BONE ON BONE

BONE *ON* BONE

An Orthopedic Surgeon's
Guide to **Avoiding Surgery** and
Healing Pain Naturally

Meredith Warner, MD

BenBella Books, Inc.
Dallas, TX

BenBella Books, Inc.
10440 N. Central Expressway
Suite 800
Dallas, TX 75231
benbellabooks.com
Send feedback to feedback@benbellabooks.com

BenBella is a federally registered trademark.

Printed in the United States of America
10 9 8 7 6 5 4 3 2 1

Library of Congress Control Number: 2023048239
ISBN 9781637745052 (hardcover)
ISBN 9781637745069 (ebook)

Editing by Alyn Wallace and Gregory Newton Brown
Copyediting by Ginny Glass
Proofreading by Becky Maines and Cape Cod Compositors, Inc.
Indexing by Debra Bowman
Text design by Aaron Edmiston
Text composition by PerfecType, Nashville, TN
Cover design by Ty Nowicki
Cover image © Adobe Stock / CLIONS
Printed by Lake Book Manufacturing

Special discounts for bulk sales are available. Please contact bulkorders@benbellabooks.com.

CONTENTS

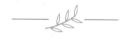

Chapter One

WHY THE WELL THEORY

I f you're holding this book, chances are good that you are in pain and your doctor has likely recommended surgery. In the United States, one in five of us has chronic pain. We suffer from some of the highest rates of the top killers—heart disease, stroke, and cancer—and from other serious conditions such as obesity and type 2 diabetes as well as Alzheimer's and other dementia-related conditions. We have very high rates of orthopedic surgeries and yet exceedingly high rates of disabilities as well.[1]

These ongoing conditions and challenges are happening even though the United States spends 18 percent of its GDP on healthcare. By 2030, the health spending share of GDP is projected to reach 19.6 percent—almost one-fifth of our total economy![2]

Despite all this spending, it's clear that our current model of care just isn't working.

THE ORTHOPEDIC COMMUNITY IS OUT OF ALIGNMENT

To be blunt about it, the medical industry has failed us. Most medical care and definitely most orthopedic care is still operating on a purely biomedical model that is reactionary. This is the basic premise of modern medicine, especially for orthopedic and musculoskeletal care: You walk in with a symptom; your doctor prescribes a test, medication, surgery, or another invasive procedure. Frequently, the doctor doesn't even perform a thorough physical examination. An MRI is often ordered, and then treatment is based on the results. The biomedical model assumes that pain or dysfunction must have a single anatomical source, which simply needs to be identified and corrected. In other words, the goal is to find a tangible reason for your "problem" and then apply a procedure or drug to "fix" it. There is no consideration of the complexity of the human body and brain with regard to your aches and pains. Physicians do not address prevention with patients. Unfortunately, this model of care is outdated and flawed, and I think it needs to be tossed.

If you have a musculoskeletal problem and are frustrated with your current care, then I hope this book will inspire you to take new action. Keep in mind that what I'm recommending here will not be what you're likely to hear in most clinics across the country. But do not be fearful. To feel better, and to improve or even reverse painful conditions that afflict you, it's not necessary to become extreme in your daily life. You don't need a private chef and a personal trainer. You don't need to monitor every bite that enters your mouth. You can still have a fun-filled life, even while becoming healthier.

What you need are just basic guidelines that will work for you in our modern world. And that's where I—and this book—come in.

A SURGEON AGAINST (SO MUCH) SURGERY

I've been treating orthopedic conditions and diseases for more than twenty years: first, on the battlefield of the streets of New Orleans, then while serving as an orthopedic surgeon during military tours in both Afghanistan and Iraq, and now in private practice. I am also honored to be clinical faculty for LSU Orthopedics. Throughout this time I have not seen much improvement in medical care. The increasing rates per capita of pain, narcotics usage, and surgeries, combined with a simultaneous increase in disability claims, demonstrate that neither evidence nor logic are prominent in the world of musculoskeletal care.

As I have grown and developed as a surgeon, clinician, and as a person, I've become more and more disenchanted with what I had been taught as the normal course of care. Yes, I'm an orthopedic surgeon, and I treat musculoskeletal conditions. And I certainly operate when that becomes necessary. In fact, I love surgery and am thrilled every time that I am able to help someone.

However, as I conduct more and more research into pain, it is obvious to me that we as orthopedic surgeons are approaching patient treatment from the wrong perspective. I have realized that a lot of the very good basic scientific research pertaining to orthopedic and rheumatologic issues, particularly nutrition research, is ignored in my field. Over time, I have learned that diet, nutrition, and lifestyle have the most significant impact on how you feel and function. In this book, I want you to learn why that is so.

To give credit where it is due, I'm encouraged that, last year, the American Board of Orthopaedic Surgery included an article for its board certification program entitled "The Role of Emotional Health in Functional Outcomes After Orthopaedic Surgery: Extending the Biopsychosocial Model to Orthopaedics." How people think and feel emotionally matters a great deal to how they feel physically! As it turns out, mindset is massively important. This is very humbling, since it is sometimes hard to accept that a patient's mindset and underlying mental health matters more than surgical skill in terms of patient outcomes.

So, progress is being made—but it is slow. And that slow progress won't help someone whose doctor has recommended potentially unnecessary surgery today.

There is no reason for you to continue to feel bad every day. There is no reason to continue to feel stiff. You can take control of your own body and health. Stay with me here, and I'll show you the results from volume after volume of studies about surgery outcomes and risks, in contrast with better outcomes from less-invasive treatments—even compared to doing nothing at all! Yes, you read that right. A multitude of studies show that changing your lifestyle—or simply doing *nothing at all*—leads to a better outcome than surgery. Even better, avoiding surgery is usually risk-free, as opposed to complication-fraught procedures. It is also generally far cheaper.

I'll add one caveat to the above: If you fall down a flight of stairs or tackle a tough ski slope and break your femur, you're going to need surgery. I perform surgeries for such work or sports accidents every week at my clinic. But in this book, we're talking not about such traumatic injuries but instead about the routine aches, pains, stiffness, muscle cramps, and immobility that "sneak up on you"—the conditions that defy you to pinpoint when and how they started. I am talking about surgeries that are indicated for what you (and your surgeon) probably consider to be the "inevitable consequences of aging"—elective surgeries that are indicated for a complaint of pain, stiffness, clicking/popping, and other subjective symptoms. I am here to tell you that most of those surgeries are probably not necessary, and that the symptoms you feel are certainly not inevitable.

Also, it has become clear with large datasets that the main reason for a surgical indication is not a symptom you have but *where you live*, combined with your surgeon's personal enthusiasm to operate.[3] In other words, your zip code determines your treatment.[4] After controlling for race, gender, education, income, and access to providers, studies show that for a given condition, the recommended treatment depends on your zip code more than anything else. How can this be? Surgeons are part of a broader community. As with all communities, groupthink tends to prevail over time. If you are unlucky enough to be in a zip code where the groupthink promotes surgery, you will be indicated for surgery. Your care also naturally depends on your own bias for preferred treatment.

Large amounts of data demonstrate that for true trauma, there is consensus on what surgery is needed. National practice is similar. For example, if you fall and break your hip, there is consensus among surgeons nationally that it should be fixed.[5] Even the type of implant and surgical techniques are similar. These sorts of surgeries are not "avoidable." But if you follow my suggestions, your outcomes from a surprise trauma surgery will be much better than they would be otherwise.

In this book, I'll lay out a preventative protocol that I've used to help countless patients avoid surgery, or recover more effectively when surgery *is* needed. You can prevent or reverse the pain in as little as three to four months, naturally, with the protocol of MEDS: Mindset, Exercise, Diet, Sleep.[6] But before we get there, let's explore some background.

WHAT ARE ORTHOPEDICS AND MUSCULOSKELETAL CARE?

The list of conditions that fall under the orthopedic-and-musculoskeletal umbrella is long. Back pain. Hip pain. Leg pain. Foot pain. Neck pain. Shoulder pain. Joint pain. Osteoarthritis. Tendinitis. Rheumatism. Autoimmune conditions. Muscular dystrophy. Neuropathy and nerve pain. Basically, any issue that involves the muscles, connective tissues, and skeleton.

Osteoarthritis, for instance, which is now considered to be a noncommunicable chronic disease (NCD), is a condition in which the cartilage covering your bones and joints becomes dysfunctional and thinner. Problems within the cells of the cartilage and with the joint capsule mean that the tissues also lack the capacity to heal themselves when damage occurs. When that happens, the cartilage loses its integrity, the bones start rubbing against each other, and the joints become painful. The pain and stiffness frequently associated with aging, such as those caused by osteoarthritis, are primarily due to constant attacks on the joint structures by chronic low-grade inflammation, oxidative stress, and other issues, all of which are preventable. In the United States, 24 percent of all adults have osteoarthritis, making it a leading cause of work disability. Other forms of arthritis, which are traditionally considered "inflammatory," include gout, rheumatoid arthritis, and lupus.[7] The fundamental problems that cause arthritis also lead to other problems with the musculoskeletal system. Mental stress, poor sleep, and toxic overload from our modern lives also contribute to everyday aches and pains within our connective tissues.

If you suffer from one of these conditions, you'll experience pain, aches, stiffness, and swelling—an unpleasant prospect. That's why you'll want to do everything possible to prevent such conditions from developing and to treat them effectively if they are already present. Unfortunately, the existing medical care model will push you toward orthopedic surgery, injections, or drugs.

AGING AND PAIN

Hardly a week passes that some patient doesn't walk into my orthopedic clinic with comments like these: "Well, I just turned forty. I guess it's all downhill from here." Or, "I'm sixty-five, so at my age, I guess I need to expect these aches and pains."

But they're wrong. Aches and pains don't necessarily accompany aging. Of course, that's not to say that people don't have pain. They do! Musculoskeletal pain—pain caused by muscles, joints, bones, or nerves—affects a huge percentage of the adult population. In fact, musculoskeletal problems are a leading cause of global disability. For many people, pain is a fact of life at one time or another. We have pain from injuries. We have aches from viruses and bacterial infections spread through the air we breathe. Even kids have pain in their legs and arms when they experience a sudden growth spurt.

Without a doubt, pain is big business for physicians and pharmaceutical companies that market pain medications. But keep in mind these medicines treat symptoms—not necessarily the actual causes of pain. It is also important to understand the relationship between pain and nociception. Nociceptors sense changes in tissue and send a signal to the brain. The brain modifies and interprets those signals, and many variables are at play. This interpretation is "pain." This is meant to indicate that there might be danger and a need for protection, but these signals can be dramatically changed and not reflect reality at all.

Instead of understanding pain as simply the biological phenomenon that it is, we seek painkillers to mask it. We are never taught the true causes of the pain. We ask surgeons for surgeries and other procedures and ask pain-management doctors for more pills rather than taking an active role in staying well. Or we let pain-management doctors escalate our dosing of opioids without question.

But taking an active role in handling pain doesn't mean over-the-counter, "harmless" pills. Although these over-the-counter drugs are typically safe when used as directed, some can create serious consequences. For example, simple meds like acetaminophen (Tylenol), laxatives, aspirin, and cold medicines can cause serious adverse effects. To be specific, in the United States, about sixty thousand people a year are hospitalized for acetaminophen overdose complications.[8]

Thousands of people also end up being treated for either GI or cardiac side effects from non-steroidal anti-inflammatory drugs (NSAIDs), like ibuprofen. So make sure you take a balanced look at the pros and cons of even over-the-counter medicines as well as those prescribed by your doctor.

Granted, time will pass—but that doesn't mean we must suffer age-related pain. The goal—certainly, my goal as an orthopedic surgeon—is to help you lengthen your health span to relate to your chronological age more closely. Some people at age ninety still feel vibrant and live pain-free like younger people at age fifty or sixty. Some thirty-year-olds are trying to get on disability because of aches and pains.

Increasing your health span is possible by paying attention to your MEDS (positive *mindset*, proper *exercise*, healthy *diet*, and restorative *sleep*). Aging-related comorbidities (heart disease, diabetes, cancer) take their toll. Changes in your tissues from chronic inflammation, oxidative stress, and toxins lead to deterioration of your organs. The decline in organ function happens over time—even without an injury or a disease. This time-related deterioration is what is currently considered aging. Believe it or not, most of your problems are from lifestyle choices. Most of them can be prevented, managed, or reversed by better choices.

THE TROUBLE WITH MRI

When you see a doctor for a pain complaint, the most common tool that will eventually indicate you for an orthopedic procedure is magnetic resonance imaging (MRI). In my opinion, MRI studies are overused and, as a result, have become diagnostic crutches. Let's take a look at what MRI does and does not show before some physician waves an MRI report in front of you with the pronouncement, "You're gonna need surgery."

Magnetic resonance imaging is an amazing and wonderful technology that literally allows physicians to look inside the body and see spots that we consider "abnormal." Following the biomedical principles of traditional medical practice, we then say that if we "fix" that spot, we will solve the problem, and your symptoms will go away. However, the findings provided by MRI studies may not, in fact, be the true source of pain.

Before you respond, "Yeah, but my MRI shows—," consider this: Landmark MRI studies of large groups of people show abnormalities in patients with no symptoms at all. That goes for MRIs showing abnormalities in the cervical spine, lumbar spine, knee, hip, and shoulder of a patient! The same "defect" that your surgeon found on your MRI and said should be fixed is probably on the MRI scans of countless people with no pain or symptoms at all.

To be clear, millions of people are walking around with rotator cuff tears, arthritis, or a torn meniscus at the knee—but they have no pain. They're enjoying full, normal function.[9] In fact, the prevalence of biomedical "abnormalities" on MRI is so common, the abnormalities are now considered to be normal.

The logical conclusion follows that the abnormality, protrusion, herniated disc, or arthritic tissue may or may not be the cause of a patient's symptoms. The symptoms may stem from other things such as chronic inflammation, poor diet, lack of exercise, or poor sleep.

That is, MRIs do not take the root cause into account. MRIs serve only to demonstrate that there is a finding, or there is something that can be pointed to as a biomedical "abnormality." In reality, the pain experienced by the patient is usually a *symptom* of another underlying condition or disease that is not going to be seen on that MRI. But some doctors simply take the easiest path to diagnosis. Rather than identify the underlying cause, they refer only to the MRI scans and routinely recommend surgery. In fact, if I order lumbar MRIs in my clinic, I can almost guarantee that there will be a finding and a possible procedure to be done.

I do not own an MRI or have a share or financial relationship with one, but many physicians do. The growth rate of MRI studies completed between 2000 and 2005 was 254 percent for nonradiologist-physician-owned MRI machines, as opposed to only 83 percent for those owned by radiologists.[10]

Procedure volumes have also grown along with the number of MRI studies completed. This is the natural result of discovering a greater number of "abnormalities" detected that thus require "fixing." A brief examination of what MRIs show—and what they don't show—will demonstrate the extent of the problem.

One of my favorite books, *American Pain* by John Temple, recounts the beginning of the opioid epidemic in the United States and the so-called pill mills. These still exist—they are just well hidden by new regulations. Two brothers created an empire by hiring some doctors and placing pharmacies inside offices within strip malls throughout the southeast United States. Government officials began to clamp down; one of the primary weapons the regulators used to stop this addiction train was to deem that prescriptions were not medically necessary.

The brothers were quite cunning and soon figured out that all that was needed was a quick MRI right before the visit to establish "medical necessity." Not only could they make more cash from the study, but they knew that each and every MRI would generate a finding that would allow them to achieve the goal of medical necessity.[11] This story shows how MRIs can be used against you—everyone in the medical community knows they will see something that can explain your pain and justify a procedure or a drug. Meanwhile, the medical literature shows that almost all findings from an MRI scan reflect a normal part of being a live, upright, biped human being.

An IBM sales consultant once quipped, "Nobody ever gets fired for buying IBM." He went on to explain that when a potential client becomes confused about which vendors to choose for new hardware, software, or business consulting, no higher-up will ever fault a decision to select an established, reputable brand. Their products and service come with a recognizable guarantee of quality.

Likewise, physicians holding an MRI showing an abnormality will be safe in recommending surgery. No insurance company will question the decision if the wording on the radiology report is correct. Furthermore, the patient and family will likely go along with that recommendation.

Everyone's happy—unless the surgery causes further damage or doesn't relieve the pain or correct the problem.

The Back: What MRIs Show—and Don't Show

Back pain is a common complaint. If you have back pain, your doctor may describe it in several ways. For example, you may be told that you have a bulging or herniated disc. If the discs bulge out too close to a nerve, the nerves running down your arms or legs can become inflamed. Or your doctor might tell you that your MRI shows that a disc is compressing a nerve root. A "pinched nerve" typically hurts somewhere other than in your back. This is because each nerve root has a region of responsibility for sensations that are sent to the brain. If that nerve root fires for any reason, the brain will interpret that as pain or something similar. The pattern of each nerve root is called a dermatome. Each dermatome has a specific pathway that is the same for all of us. For example, if the top of the foot and the side of your leg hurts, that might be due to an L5 nerve root issue, because that is part of its dermatome.

But here's the question some patients ask: "What if back surgery provides some short-term relief? Then wouldn't the surgery still be worth the risks, costs, and the recovery period?" The short answer is of course that if you know the surgery risks and decide to have surgery anyway, then that's your choice. However, for several reasons, most patients believe in their hearts that they need surgery. They are in pain, for instance, and their doctors told them there was a finding on the MRI that is the reason for that pain. I can't tell you how many people I have treated successfully with nonoperative methods for back pain whose first statement was that their doctor had recommended surgery. Don't make the choice for surgery, however, based solely on your MRI results!

There are many studies that demonstrate the lack of usefulness of MRI for diagnosing back pain. MRI findings on spinal MRI studies are not predictive of back pain in the future. Disc bulges and other findings like arthritis are seen in elite athletes who play at a high level but who do not experience pain. There are many papers demonstrating that bulging discs, degeneration, herniated discs, and many other "abnormalities" are clearly normal and should be expected for upright human beings who are still alive. The data is clear that the mere presence of these findings does not mean that they are the reasons for the pain or stiffness.

Abnormalities on MRIs must be strictly correlated with age and with any other clinical signs and symptoms before surgery is recommended as the best treatment.[12] Numerous studies have warned that if there is such a large chance that there will be an abnormal finding on MRI, with or without symptoms, then it is dangerous to predicate a surgical decision on that finding.[13]

The Shoulder: What MRIs Show—and Don't Show

Shoulder pain is another common orthopedic complaint. Your two shoulder joints each consist of three bones: the clavicle, the scapula, and the humerus. These shoulder joints give you the capacity to rotate your arms in many different directions—in case you want to climb a tree, toss a two-year-old over your head, or swing a golf club. The rotator cuff is a group of four muscles that stabilize the ball (humerus) in its shallow socket (the glenoid of the scapula) during motion. Rotator cuff surgeries are one of the most common surgeries in the world.

A rotator cuff injury is typically thought of as a strain or tear of the muscles or tendons around those shoulder bones. Most often, you are told that you can avoid shoulder injuries if you pay attention to the position of your arm when you're moving it. Extending your arm so far back that you can't see it in your peripheral vision, for instance, often leads to damage. However, most shoulder pain happens for no apparent reason. Today, science has shown us that most shoulder pain is probably due to the same forces that cause dementia, heart disease, diabetes, and other NCDs. What you need to know is that rotator cuff tears are very common and are often seen in people with absolutely no shoulder pain. Be mindful of the number of abnormalities visualized in the shoulders of people without any pain or dysfunction before you commit to a surgery.[14]

The Knee: What MRIs Show—and Don't Show

Your knee, situated between the femur and tibia bones, mimics a door hinge. It moves backward and forward, not side to side. Osteoarthritis is a disease of the whole joint, and you should not forget the other structures beyond the bone and cartilage. There is a joint capsule with a synovial lining, and there are ligaments on both the inside and outside of the joint. Synovial linings exist around all joints and some tendons. Think of this like a deflated water balloon that holds the joint. The inside of that balloon is called the synovial lining. This is where a lot of the inflammatory proteins are produced. Most arthritic joints have thick synovial linings. There are multiple tendons that connect muscles above and below the knee, and then there are the menisci and several smaller ligaments responsible for connecting these cushion-like structures to the knee itself. The knee is a very common source of pain and knee replacements are a very common surgery in the United States. Knee arthroscopy, a surgery during which the surgeon will use a tool equipped with fiber optics to visualize the inside of a joint and another tool that is inserted to perform any tissue treatment, is even more common.

Surgery for the knee is often predicated on imaging findings, together with subjective complaints of pain, stiffness, and dysfunction. But, again, we have a problem with false positives provided by MRIs.[15] Indeed, MRIs with "abnormal" findings do not necessarily show the causes of knee pain. Almost all of the individuals in a group of studies had knee abnormalities—but no symptoms, no pain! Clearly, something else is going on here—something to do with cellular metabolism and mitochondrial function, none of which have a finding on an MRI.

Similar investigations have been done for MRI studies of hips, hands, feet, and other parts of the body. In all cases, there are large percentages of people with abnormalities on imaging, but no symptoms.[16] In my opinion, such studies reveal the flaws in the biomedical method that we normally follow in orthopedics.

Just because an MRI shows that you have an abnormality, deformity, tear, or degenerative tissue, you and your physician should not jump to the conclusion that the irregular finding is the cause of your pain. Consequently, you shouldn't automatically accept the fact that you need surgery to remove, replace, or repair your defective body part.

Consider the natural remedies in the rest of this book as your treatment plan. Should you and your surgeon decide that you still require surgical intervention, hopefully, you will have a much better recovery by following the protocols I will give you. However, it is my sincere goal to empower you to prevent pain and avoid surgery with basic, evidence-based, fundamental lifestyle principles.

THE PROBLEM WITH SPECIALISTS AND CONFLICT

In the musculoskeletal field, specialization is a problem. Physicians often specialize in only one body part—spines, shoulder rotator cuff repairs, hip replacements, knee replacements, hands, or feet. Often these specialists seem to forget that a single body part belongs to an entire human being. I have a resident who makes the joke that he will specialize in treating the second toe on Wednesdays.

Conflicted referral systems add to these difficulties. Physician friends may refer to one another based only on the fact that they were on the same high school football team. Insurance companies have their own network of approved physicians and specialists; usually this means that those physicians accept less money per visit in exchange for the volume of referrals. Co-owners of clinics, surgical centers, hospitals, and testing and screening centers also have referral networks. Hospitals have their own network of doctors with privileges at their facilities; these physicians are not allowed to refer outside of the hospital's network. This means that the patient has no control over their care.

More conflicts happen that may affect your care. Financial incentives come from Big Pharma, medical equipment companies, and the food industry. These companies sponsor research studies. They "invest" in the growth of medical knowledge through grants, scholarships, and sponsorships of research activities by medical schools and hospitals. Often, these sponsorship dollars are not paid directly to physicians. Instead, they're routed indirectly through nonprofits and foundations controlled by board members from the same special-interest groups. A key study published in the *New England Journal of Medicine* found that only 71 percent of the doctors disclosed that they had received payments. For payments that were directly related to the topic of their presentation at the meeting, 79 percent provided disclosure. When considering *indirect* payments (for example, a payment routed through a nonprofit foundation), the disclosure rate fell to only 50 percent.[17]

Why didn't more physicians disclose such payments? Their three top reasons were, firstly, that they considered the payment unrelated to the topic of the presentation (39 percent); secondly, that they "misunderstood" the disclosure requirements (14 percent); and thirdly, that the payment was actually disclosed, but mistakenly omitted from the program (11 percent)![18] At the annual meeting of the American Academy of Orthopaedic Surgeons, there's only a 50 percent rate of disclosures by physicians making presentations at the conference—despite the fact the annual meeting is heavily scrutinized

Still, zipped lips! (You can only imagine the low rates of disclosing these payments during smaller medical meetings around the country with less scrutiny and investigation.) Considering heavy penalties, fines, and loss of reputation, why would physicians take the risk of failing to report these payments?

The leading reason cited is that the physician considered his or her presentation topic unrelated to the payment they've received. Those who decide not to disclose such payments often simply refuse to acknowledge a link between their research or recommendations and influence from special interest groups. Instead, they insist that their presentations related to surgeries, medications, or other treatments are intended only to contribute to the body of medical knowledge and have no influence on their patient decisions or research findings. This position among surgeons may, however, be changing, since the current climate places enormous pressure on physicians to be more ethical and transparent than our elected legislators.

So, what's the government doing about such lack of transparency among physicians? Action in 2007 by the Department of Justice somewhat improved the situation. The five companies that sell most of the hip and knee implants in the United States averted criminal prosecution over illegal kickbacks by agreeing to federal monitoring and promising to comply with new procedures and policies. In 2008, such kickbacks declined. Then when the eighteen-month agreements expired in March 2009, four of these five companies entered into corporate integrity agreements (CIAs) with the Department of Health and Human Services. At the time of this writing, these CIAs have now expanded to include thirty companies.

Was your own physician caught up in these illegal activities? Probably not. According to the study, approximately one thousand physicians who received payments in 2007 represent only about 4 percent of the orthopedic surgeons in the United States. So, odds are your local orthopedic surgeon has been transparent with you.

Scandals continue to surface regarding published articles in reputable, well-known journals. For example, consider the issues around Alzheimer's studies. A study originally published in *Nature* back in 2006 was revealed in 2022 to contain some falsified data. To make matters worse, research on Alzheimer's conducted since that point was based on that same falsified data, with authors citing the original study thousands of times.[19]

Another scandal recently surfaced involving the *New England Journal of Medicine*. This journal hid the fact that the authors of a 1967 article assuring that sugar in our diets created no harm was actually funded by the sugar industry.[20]

Another example involves a newly published study that shows no evidence that serotonin levels are abnormal in depressed individuals.[21] Yet many of the antidepressant makers base their drugs on the theory that increasing serotonin will improve the condition. For example, many people take selective serotonin reuptake inhibitors (SSRIs). Why would patients need these if their serotonin levels are not relevant to the disorder?

Finally, let's not overlook scandals in the orthopedic world. A few years ago, investigations revealed that a large device company had paid surgeons to publish an article stating that a certain product improved fusion rates in spine surgery. These studies were published by *The Spine Journal*, causing the publication to commit to extensive changes in their manuscript-review procedure and policies for disclosing conflicts of interest.[22]

Fortunately, the medical industry investigates and reports on its own failures.[23] It has become standard practice in medical journals to require authors to disclose their relationships with industry. But these requirements vary between journals and often lack specific criteria and explanations. As a result, disclosures don't consistently reveal ties between authors and industry.[24]

BIAS TO FOLLOW PROTOCOLS, RATHER THAN BUILD PATIENT PROFILES

For decades, medical schools have taught physicians to follow algorithms for treatment based on "evidence," rather than treating a patient by looking at their entire profile and personalizing their treatment. For example, you complain of tingling in your arm, hand, and fingers. The physician will do a nerve-conduction test. If that's positive, they'll diagnose you with carpal tunnel syndrome and schedule surgery. They may never discuss with you the underlying cause of your carpal tunnel or suggest ways to prevent similar problems in the future.

Currently, surgical societies have also published guidelines regarding certain problems or diagnoses. Many insurance companies now use artificial intelligence (AI) systems based on these guidelines to build an algorithm that either approves or denies a request for service. As an example, if I have a patient who needs a knee brace to take the pressure off the medial (inside) compartment of her arthritic knee, I must request permission.

Why is requesting permission a problem? Well, for starters, in my note, I must state certain things, such as confirming that the patient is not obese and is still active. And if the radiology report does not state specifically that "more than 50 percent of the joint space remains" and further state that the grade of arthritis is "Kellgren-Lawrence stage 1 or 2," then the computer will deny the patient's brace. So, this limits my ability to provide nonsurgical care for that patient.

That brings us back to the model taught in medical school:

1. Listen to the symptoms.
2. Find the cause.
3. Fix the cause.

Only rarely do health-care professionals and insurance companies focus on prevention. The system is designed to ignore diet, mindset, sleep, and natural remedies.

Like the restrictions in requesting permission for patient treatments, physicians must select the "cause" from a limited list of options. If an orthopedic surgeon has a patient with knee pain, the list of causes will only include anatomic structures in the knee. Other causes are excluded from the list. No mention of fascial tightness at the lumbosacral fascia or hip. No mention about psychological variables like depression or anxiety. No mention of oxidative stress, chronic inflammation, or other systemic and diet-based sources of pain. None of these other plausible reasons appear in the "causes" list. I can think of no clearer explanation than this saying: "If all you have is a hammer, everything looks like a nail."

Any other alternative or natural treatments—such as those involving diet, exercise, sleep, meditation, hot and cold exposure, acupuncture, and so on—are considered experimental. The word *experimental* is code for "we won't pay for that." Many physicians simply refuse to investigate nontraditional views about natural treatments and therapies. Worse, most of these methods to make people feel better are not covered by any insurance plan I've ever seen.

Of course—and as noted earlier—surgery is clearly warranted in some cases, such as when you break a femur in a traumatic car accident. But the body itself, with proper nutrients and care, can prevent, improve, or potentially heal many other serious conditions such as diabetes, fibromyalgia, neuropathy, heart attacks, strokes, Alzheimer's, Parkinson's, and cancer. The same is true for problems associated with autoimmune disorders, connective tissue disorders, osteoarthritis, and other problems causing common pain and stiffness.

EGOS TIED TO OUTCOMES

As in any field, from sales to sports, certain professionals see themselves as superstars. Physicians are no different. Some seem to communicate that attitude with their body language, bedside manner, or biased recommendations.

Sometimes, the ego-outcome link is so strong that physicians try to lower expectations with patients and their families. Before going into surgery, they make statements like these: "This tear is the worst I've seen. I'm just hoping that the surgery will fix it. We've got about a 60–70 percent chance this will work." Then if the outcome disappoints the patient, the physician can always say that they did the best with such a terrible injury or difficult circumstance.

In our modern times, when surgeries don't go well, physicians often don't even see the patient for follow-up. Instead, they refer them immediately to a pain-management doctor, who gives narcotics or injections. In my experience, this is becoming the standard of care. That is, at the first postoperative visit, the patient is referred immediately to pain management. This happens even before the bones or ligaments have healed! The underlying implication is that there will still always be pain, so what was "fixed"?

Even for wonderfully compassionate and competent doctors, their egos swell or suffer depending on patient outcomes. If all goes well, they take a victory lap. If things go wrong and a patient dies or has a bad outcome, they can become overwhelmed by guilt; in fact, the suicide rate for physicians (28 to 40 per 100,000) is twice that of the rest of the population.[25]

DIFFICULT, PUSHY PATIENTS

For a variety of reasons, patients themselves may push for a more radical, invasive procedure than necessary. For starters, solving their health problem with lifestyle changes such as diet and exercise can be difficult. It's hard to overcome a victim mindset or to escape the clutches of learned helplessness.

Some patients want to eat what they want to eat—no matter how many of their aches and pains come from poor nutrition. Similarly, patients sometimes hate to exercise—no matter how much they know about the value of exercise to build endurance, strengthen bones, improve mood, build muscle mass, and protect the brain.

Sometimes patients berate the evidence that shows how poor sleep habits affect their bodies in myriad negative ways. So, they continue to deprive themselves of sleep—critical time during which the body repairs its own tissues. The leading group of these sleep-deprived people? Physicians!

And let's face it: Some physicians—who can also end up being patients themselves—are poor role models for making lifestyle changes of any kind. Many are out of shape themselves. We've known cardiologists who do not control their weight. We've known gastrologists suffering from acid reflux who don't control how much spicy or toxic food they eat. We've known dermatologists who don't protect themselves from the sun. We've known orthopedic doctors who've had to have knee replacements because their frame cannot bear their weight. And don't get me started about the doctors I know who still smoke.

It feels hypocritical for physicians to recommend lifestyle changes to patients when they cannot or do not make such changes themselves.

So, with pushy patients, physicians may find themselves on the defensive without a proper pitch. That is, pointing out the patient's obesity as a probable cause of aching knees can create patient rage. Mentioning depression or negativism as a probable cause of low-back pain may generate patient skepticism. Probing patients about ridding themselves of job-related stress or reducing their workloads can enrage people who insist they're irreplaceable at work.

For many patients, asking for surgery or a pill to correct a problem can be much easier than making lifestyle changes. And if these patients don't get the surgery, procedure, or pill they want or think they need, they can always go "doctor shopping" until they find someone who will accommodate them. For many physicians, the only "doctor-like" recommendation they can offer is a pill, procedure, or surgery. After all, in the physician's way of reasoning,

Aunt Ida or Cousin Max can surely discuss diet and exercise with them over Sunday lunch.

If the patient feels vengeful after a physician balks at giving them what they want, they can always threaten to post negative comments on social media sites like Yelp or write bad reviews on the doctor's own website. We all expect this to occur when we don't fill a requested narcotics prescription. Unfortunately, physicians are not allowed to reply to negative comments because this is prohibited by federal privacy laws.

THE BIGGER PICTURE: CONSIDER THE CONFLICTS OF INTEREST IN ALL CORNERS

In his recent book *Life Force*, Tony Robbins quotes Marcia Angell—physician, author, and the first female editor in chief of the *New England Journal of Medicine*: "Over the past two decades the pharmaceutical industry has moved very far from its original high purpose of discovering and producing useful new drugs. Now [it's] primarily a marketing machine to sell new drugs of dubious benefit."

According to the latest data available, the US pharma market in 2020 was $534.21 billion. The global market in 2021 was $1,482 billion. So, the pharmaceutical companies have power and opportunity to reward physicians and hospitals to administer their drugs. Grant money can build new hospital wings and cover the cost of the latest equipment. Medical device companies have power and opportunity to do the same for hospitals and medical schools.

Big Pharma also has considerable influence over total health-care policy—at the state and federal government level. These companies can influence FDA rulings and policies. For example, currently the FDA won't allow some natural remedies while they have approved lab-grown chicken meat from a culture for human consumption. Pharmaceutical companies spend billions annually lobbying Congress to pass or modify government regulations in favor of their industry.[26]

These companies also have astronomical annual marketing budgets for reaching doctors and consumers directly to advertise specific drugs for specific conditions. (The public is now familiar with the Purdue lawsuit and settlement for intentionally deceiving doctors on OxyContin's safety record.) Many ads end by encouraging consumers to "ask your doctor if this drug is appropriate for you." Additionally, they send pharmaceutical reps directly to physicians, clinics, and hospitals to give away samples of their products.

Doctors vie with each other to make presentations about their work and outcomes to pharmaceutical or medical-device companies. Consequently, these physicians find themselves with opportunities to land grants for pet research projects, receive honoraria for speeches to corporate audiences, and land consulting contracts or advisory positions.[27]

Finally, consider the influence of insurance companies. In addition to grants, scholarships, and sponsorships at medical-industry conferences, they have ultimate power in saying yes or no to a physician's recommended treatment. The insurance company's utilization reviewer never even sees a patient. Their only criteria for approving or declining a treatment are test results and the computer algorithm. A physician's opinion only occasionally matters.

To change the traditional medical industry, then, you as a patient will need to lead the charge. Consider this book as your guide. Educate yourself about natural remedies, treatments, and therapies—those that are nonsurgical, noninvasive, and less costly. Sure, most of us are covered by some form of insurance. But in addition to our ever-rising insurance premiums, on average, patients spend $1,200 annually on prescription drugs—and that's not even counting over-the-counter medications.[28] These drug costs, along with other treatment costs, are covered by the insurance companies and then passed on to you through rising insurance premiums. Despite this, there's still no reward or incentive from insurance companies for staying healthy. So don't expect any insurance help with the natural treatments you'll find recommended in this book.

Remember: it's up to you as a patient to take the lead in driving toward the health care you need and deserve!

DOES SURGERY SOLVE ALL PROBLEMS?

Tom, a fifty-five-year-old man, came to see me with shoulder pain that had profoundly altered his life. He used to be an avid golfer, but now could only putt. He had initially developed shoulder pain a couple of years prior to seeing me. The MRI revealed a rotator cuff tear, and he was indicated for surgery a month later. No other treatment had been offered to him. One year on, because he was not doing well and still had pain, another MRI was ordered. This one showed another tear, but now the muscle looked weak, and the tendon had pulled from the bone. Another surgery was performed. About six months after that, Tom was suffering from even worse pain and had now become very stiff. The third MRI showed another retear; the retraction was larger, and the muscle looked worse. This is when he came to see me for my opinion. I discovered that he had very limited motion in certain directions and his posterior shoulder muscles were exceedingly weak. I put lidocaine into the shoulder capsule and retested him. Once he had the numbing medicine in the shoulder, beneath the acromion inside of an inflamed sac of tissue, he was able to move his shoulder a bit more and had far less pain. This gave me hope that my therapy team could work on his pain with a very focused rehabilitation and mobilization program.

Contrast Tom's situation with that of Jennifer. Jennifer is a sixty-five-year-old female and came to see me with shoulder pain. An MRI demonstrated full thickness and retracted tears of her rotator cuff. Knowing the data on the high retear rate after surgery for such problems, and knowing that the underlying pain was probably more from a lack of coordinated and conditioned muscle units around the shoulder, I moved forward with a physical therapy protocol, along with natural supplements to manage chronic inflammation. Jennifer had complete resolution of her pain and near full range of motion after about five months of therapy. Yet her tear was still present. This is an example of how the problem, as defined by an MRI, may not really be the source of the symptoms. Worse, when surgery is performed, it is often not curative and sometimes can make things a little worse.

Although hip replacement surgery is a good option with generally positive outcomes, it is not without its own problems and risks. And I'm not talking about risks such as difficulty with the anesthesia or accidental mishap. I'm referring to how things can "go downhill" after hip-replacement surgery. More than 370,000 hip replacements were performed in the United States in 2014 with the main reason being osteoarthritis. This grew to 450,000 in 2020, and there is no end in sight to this growth. The authors of a review of total hip replacements found that "symptoms are not reliably associated with the degree of structural disease on imaging."[29]

For example, researchers found that despite improvements in patients who had total hip replacements, patients were more sedentary, slept worse, and performed less physical activity two years afterward. Despite successful surgery to alleviate pain and improve their walking, then, the patients did not change their behavior afterward. The authors of the study concluded that surgery by itself might not produce "a more physically active lifestyle."[30] The researchers went on to point out that health-care providers should consider other models of care for patients having a hip replacement, such as patient education about the dangers of sitting too long and the value of getting more physical activity.

You have probably heard of the placebo effect. This is very important with regard to mindset. However, what you may not know is that the placebo effect is especially strong in surgery. Scientists report that one in three people experience the placebo effect.[31] That is, they feel better after the pseudo pill or fake surgery at least 30 percent of the time.

Studies on sham surgeries are eye-opening. A sham procedure is when a patient goes into the operating room, has anesthesia, is positioned, draped, and has incisions. What they don't have is the actual surgery. When results have been compared between people who had surgery for an orthopedic condition against those that had sham surgery, the nonsurgical groups fared the same or better than the surgical groups.

A plethora of studies support this sham surgery/placebo effect. In a review of the literature on sham surgery in orthopedics, Adriaan Louw and colleagues looked at six randomized controlled trials involving 277 subjects. The researchers rated all six studies as very good on methodological quality. Their investigation demonstrated that "sham surgery in orthopedics was as effective as actual surgery in reducing pain and improving disability."[32]

In essence, we've been mired down in that biomedical model that says surgery delivers the best outcome. Not true. If sham surgeries are as effective as actual surgeries, we must not be addressing the true cause of pain and disability, right?

More and more studies demonstrate that the number one factor for surgical outcomes is the preoperative and perioperative mindset of the patient. (The perioperative period includes the operative phase, the actual procedure, and postoperative care.) That is, when accounting for all other variables in a patient's history or profile, if the patient has depression or anxiety, the outcomes are worse than those enjoyed by patients with a positive outlook. Furthermore, there is of course abundant data in the world of psychology relating a positive mindset to the experience of pain.

The critical connection between a positive mindset about chronic pain or favorable treatment and outcomes has been examined in the scientific literature for more than twenty years. Study after study has suggested that a positive outlook will lengthen life, reduce illness, control pain, improve performance, and reduce deaths from all causes. One more point you should know: diet also plays a very large role in mental health and overall mindset.

LIFESTYLE MEDICINE IS A MOVEMENT

Given all the above, what treatments should you as a patient with pain or other symptoms consider? I think the answer is clear: Natural therapies and treatments. Diets that decrease chronic inflammation and pain. Lifestyle changes that lead to prevention.

Lifestyle medicine has become a movement in the last four decades. You've probably noticed that, simply by participating in conversations at work, in your neighborhood, or at a sports event. People have a growing awareness of the power of lifestyle changes to prevent the most common chronic diseases—and even reverse their progression.

And the best news: These lifestyle changes do not involve drugs or surgery. In fact, in this book, you'll see why we suggest that these lifestyle changes affect many processes in the body—not just one specific condition, ache, or pain. These process and changes all interrelate. The same things that will reduce your pain and make you feel better and able to do more will also make your heart, brain, GI tract, kidneys, and liver healthier.

KNOWING BETTER IS NOT THE SAME AS DOING BETTER

To make a lasting change in your own health, you must commit to change. Yes, you have to *decide* to make healthy choices to prevent and reverse diseases and conditions. The challenge may seem daunting at first. But usually, it only takes 60–90 days for real change to begin. Then most people wonder why they ever lived any differently!

My lifestyle protocol for feeling better rests on four pillars of good health: a positive health *mindset*, moderate *exercise, diet* (nutrition really matters), and restorative *sleep*. The rest of this book will elaborate on each of these critical components that lead to transformative health and an extended health span as you age. Because those four considerations are so crucial to your long-term well-being, latch on to this acronym to keep them in the forefront of your mind. Granted, we're altering the typical meaning of MEDS.

M = Mindset: positive outlook, less stress, social interactions to provide support and happiness, having a health mindset

E = Exercise: moderate exercise, including resistance training

D = Diet: time-restricted eating and the Mediterranean lifestyle

S = Sleep: establishing a solid circadian rhythm and routine

Instead of the typical tray of daily pills, let mindset, exercise, diet, and sleep become your personal MEDS list. And trust me: I'm not going to debate a passel of specialists about which of these four is most critical. My goal is just to help you recall them every single day of your life to eliminate aches and pains without a prescription and transform your health for the long term.

My approach is based on an extensive amount research and experience with nonsurgical care for common musculoskeletal problems. Once I realized how little traditional methods helped with the pain my patients reported to me, I developed other ways to help them. This involved changing my perspective and thinking more holistically. It seemed to me that most of the conditions I was seeing were caused by the same things that caused other chronic health conditions: chronic inflammation, oxidative stress, and other fundamental metabolic problems. The basic role of nutrition also became painfully obvious, even though nutrition was not taught in medical school and certainly not in residency. I have learned so much that can help you, and I want to share this knowledge.

Now I'm not going to lie to you and say all these changes are easy-peasy and that they will eliminate any and all of your pain day after tomorrow. But after adopting these lifestyle changes, you will see dramatic improvement over time—typically within 60–90 days. Remember that it took the food industry and modern life years to make you unhealthy, so be patient as you reverse their work.

YOU NEED NOT BE DEFINED BY YOUR DISEASE OR CONDITION

You frequently hear friends refer to themselves by their condition as easily as they drop their name. In the same way that they might say "Hi, I'm John Smith, VP of marketing," they might refer to "my blood pressure," "my arthritis," or "my heart condition" as a reason or limitation in doing this or that. You'll hear them say things like, "With my heart condition, I always take the elevator." Or, "My bad back won't let me play tennis." It's as if they're assuming their physical condition has become a permanent part of their existence.

A first step in moving toward a new lifestyle is to separate these two things in your mind: your body, and a disease or condition. You are not the condition or disease; it doesn't have to determine your destiny.

Your body represents a complex organism all by itself. So far, scientists have estimated that:

- The average human body is made up of more than 37 trillion cells.
- The bacteria cells in our gut total about 100 to 400 trillion.
- You have approximately 70 million cell duplications every day.
- The average adult's heart beats more than one hundred thousand times each day.
- Your body experiences a billion chemical reactions per second per cell. That is 37 billion trillion reactions every second.
- You have twenty-two thousand genes—give or take a few, depending on how they mutate.
- You have 650 muscles to keep in shape.
- You have 206 bones in your body (unless a few have been replaced by implants).
- Your bones are four times stronger than concrete and stronger even than some steel. Bone can repair itself as well, while concrete and steel cannot.
- Your eyes have more than 2 million working parts.
- The digestive tract can run up to thirty feet in the average adult. (About sixty tons of food passes through in a lifetime.)
- Blood flows from your heart through your entire body and back to your heart in about forty-five seconds.
- Information travels through your brain from synapse to synapse at about 270 miles per hour.

Rest assured, then, that neither you nor your body can be described or evaluated by one specific condition. Nix that thinking so you can grasp the vision of how little you need to change to revamp your systems and improve how you feel.

THE BIG BENEFITS OF THESE LIFESTYLE CHANGES

You will achieve some or all of the following:

- Eliminate aches and pains from joints and muscles within months
- Boost your energy and mood without depending on caffeine, alcohol, or other stimulants
- Increase your flexibility, strength, muscle mass, and overall mobility to participate in favorite pastimes, hobbies, sports, and family activities
- Improve stamina for tasks requiring endurance
- Increase your bone density to prevent fractures
- Speed up your metabolism and lose excess weight
- Get better, more restorative sleep
- Reduce your risks of cognitive decline and related diseases such as Alzheimer's and Parkinson's
- Reduce your risk of all forms of cancer
- Reduce your risk of stroke
- Prevent type 2 diabetes
- Improve your heart function and reduce the risk of heart disease
- Reverse some autoimmune diseases
- Prolong your vitality and health span—the years you spend without disease or disability
- Enjoy the peace of mind and lower stress that a healthy body delivers
- Avoid costly medications and procedures that merely manage symptoms, rather than treat the cause or prevent them

PROTOCOL FOR MAKING LIFESTYLE CHANGES EASY

This lifestyle change is designed to help you feel good, happy, and powerful in your own body. Most of my patients simply want to be able to play with their grandkids on the floor and get up easily. They want to wake up and not feel completely stiff. They want to be able to enjoy their work, family, friends, and life. Most are not worried about adding a couple of years at the end of their lives—at least not yet. The Well Theory Protocol is really made for you to enhance your life at this moment. The myriad of health benefits that come with this protocol are simply extras for you. As I mentioned earlier, changes in habits don't come easy. On the other hand, lifestyle changes need not be complex. So let me give you a protocol for moving in this healthier direction with MEDS:

1. **Adopt the right mindset.** Learning new information isn't enough. You have to make up your mind that you *want* to make proven changes, that you *need* to make changes, that you *can* make changes. If you think these changes will be based on emotion, you're exactly right. You have to rev up how you feel about making these smart, logical changes.

2. **Forget everything you "know."** That includes what you might know about weight loss, muscle mass, strength training, good foods, bad foods, and so forth. In the rest of the book, you'll learn about studies that will likely revamp your thinking about what works and what doesn't work. Things don't have to be as complicated as you think.

3. **Forget your MRI.**

4. **Get a second opinion!** If the first physician neglects to tell you about options other than surgery or medications to correct whatever ails you, find one a bit more open-minded. Remember that your zip code determines treatment choices.

5. **Improve your sleep habits.** Make sure they're aligned with the circadian clock. Get up and go to bed at the same time every day. Reduce your stress and kick the sleep aids. Sleeping better forms the foundation of the Well Theory Protocol.

6. **Adopt time-restricted eating.** We'll explain much more about this later, particularly about the importance of matching your eating schedule with your circadian rhythm, but for now, just keep in mind that you're not going to be eating around the clock anymore.

7. **Modify your diet so that you're gradually moving to a Mediterranean lifestyle**,

8. **Move. Walk.** Exercise in any way you like, *but* aim to keep your blood flowing and your internal processes in good working order. Work on keeping the muscle you have—it helps to reduce pain.

9. **Connect with people socially.** Mental stress is a primary cause of chronic inflammation, leading to pain. Work and a meaningful purpose in life prevent cognitive decline. Having supporting relationships at work and in your personal life keeps depression at bay, adds fun and satisfaction, and helps you maintain a positive outlook.

In effect, with these lifestyle changes—MEDS = mindset, exercise, diet, and sleep—and other natural therapies and treatments, you will rejuvenate your entire body. In the following chapters, we will take a look at some of the science supporting the principle of MEDS and go through each part of the protocol in turn. Then we will look at some of those therapies and natural treatments to add to your armory before examining some key questions to ask your doctor at your visit. In the two appendices, you'll find detailed information about supplements and common ailments that can be treated or managed without having to go to the doctor in the first place. My protocol—MEDS—will help you live a fully functional, fulfilled, pain-free, productive, independent, joyful life into your eighties, nineties, or even past one hundred years.

So, are you ready to give it a go?

Chapter Two

WHY YOUR BODY LOVES ANTIOXIDANTS AND HATES CHRONIC INFLAMMATION

The natural healing force within each one of us is the greatest force in getting well.

—Hippocrates

When you walk into a clinic with symptoms, physicians have a tendency to reach for the knife, the needle, or the pill bottle. After all, it takes much more time to sit down and talk with you about simple, natural treatments and remedies available to correct what's ailing you:

- Stop eating food that causes inflammation.
- Eat more that aids your system to function properly.
- Sleep long enough so your body has time to repair damaged cells.
- Exercise enough so your muscles and joints get stronger and more flexible.
- Avoid large glucose spikes and insulin resistance.

- Reduce unnecessary mental stress.
- Think about the positive relationships in your life and be optimistic.

Those recommendations often turn into long discussions in my clinic because they're significant to long-term wellness. And like Jane, some people need a long, long discussion!

Jane, a thirty-year-old obese woman with type 2 diabetes, came to my clinic, complaining of hip pain. So, I started to describe an anti-inflammatory diet to her: "The first thing you need to know about this diet is to cut out processed red meat."

She looked at me blankly for a moment, and then asked, "So what actually counts as red meat?" This is not an uncommon question. Many people lack the understanding I would like them to have regarding nutrition. Some of this is by design, of course. Perhaps you recall one of the greatest marketing campaigns of all time. The pork industry rolled out the slogan "Pork—the other white meat" in 1987. Pork was pitched to the public as a good alternative to red meat. The USDA, however, classifies pork as a red meat. The program promoted pork as a lean meat, and sales grew.

With patients like Jane, the Mediterranean-lifestyle eating plan can turn into discussions as long as those TV series running fifteen seasons, with eighteen episodes per! But a caring doctor *will* connect and take the time to explain.

Warning: This chapter may be toxic to your ability to remain uninformed. We're going deeper on the *whys* and *hows* behind the *whats* of nutrition. Your health, functionality, pain control, and happiness depend on what you put in your mouth. So, in this chapter, you'll learn how the body processes food that either improves, restores, or damages your health.

WHAT IS CHRONIC INFLAMMATION?

First, let's quickly discuss inflammation in general, and why it is important for your body. Infections and injuries trigger your body's immune system response. The system consists of innate and adaptive immune cells. The first to the scene are members of the innate immune system. This includes neutrophils and natural killer cells. These cells recognize pathogenic or damaged cells as alien and destroy them with little weapons packets. These packets are held by immune cells and are filled with oxidative substances that kill the bacteria or virus.

Next, a clean-up phase happens. Immune cells called macrophages produce free radicals as they fight off invading germs and help to remove the debris created by the innate system. As already stated, these free radicals can damage healthy cells, leading to inflammation. Some of the reactive oxygen species produced by the mitochondria act to signal the innate immune system. Eventually, you will engage your adaptive immune system and utilize antibodies to fight off pathogens. As you can see, inflammation is normal and good in these situations.

Now consider *temporary* inflammation. Recall some injury you've had where part of your body swelled, turned red, felt hot, and hurt. This response happens even with a paper cut. The oxidative stress and activity of the immune cells triggered cause mild, temporary inflammation, which actually helps if you're trying to fight off a pathogen or to heal an injury. By inducing more blood flow, more molecules enter the area to assist with the healing process. This brings swelling. The redness is usually from increased blood flow to the area. Pain begins with inflammatory substances irritating nerve endings and from the damage itself. The sensation of heat is also from increased blood. Incidentally, fever is the elevation of the core body set-point of temperature, which takes place as another defense mechanism. Raising the body's temperature creates an inhospitable environment for bacteria and viruses. Immune mediators (pyrogens) trigger a part of the hypothalamus to elevate the temperature. Prostaglandins are also important here.

Inflammation is particularly relevant to daily aches and pains as the connective tissues' extracellular matrix (ECM) harbors much of the immune system. These cells sit in fascia and simply wait for signals to deploy. That is why so many autoimmune disorders cause body pains.

Prostaglandins are formed from substances in the cell membrane. The membrane phospholipids, typically derived from omega-6 fatty acids replete in the American diet, are converted to arachidonic acid by the enzyme phospholipase A2. Arachidonic acid is converted to prostaglandins by the cyclooxygenase enzymes (COX1, COX2). This is why steroids and NSAIDs can reduce fever and inflammation. They block phospholipase A2 and COX1/2 respectively.

Your defense system, however, doesn't always work so smoothly. Acute inflammation can become deadly when it stays on "high alert." Sometimes the oxidative stress just triggers more inflammation, which produces more free radicals, and which then leads to more oxidative stress. This whole process can eventually become an endless, vicious cycle lasting for weeks, months, or years.

This long-lasting, low-grade inflammation occurs as a result of several unhealthy lifestyle choices: smoking, poor diet, alcohol overindulgence, lack of exercise, stress, exposure to pollution, poor sleep, and metabolic dysfunction. Having a large amount of advanced glycation end products (AGEs) can also cause this. Symptoms of chronic inflammation include all sorts:

- Abdominal pain
- Chest pain
- Fatigue, insomnia
- Depression, anxiety
- Fever
- Joint pain or stiffness
- Skin rash
- Weight gain or loss
- Brain fog and memory loss
- Poor emotional resilience during stress
- Neuropathic pain

Over longer periods of time, chronic inflammation can lead to a number of diseases and conditions:

- Cancer
- Heart disease
- Stroke

- Neurodegenerative disorders
- Dementia
- Arthritis
- Tendinitis and other connective tissue problems
- Type 2 diabetes
- Asthma
- High blood pressure
- IBS
- Psoriasis
- Skin disorders
- Constipation-based conditions (diverticulosis, hemorrhoids, varicose veins, colon cancer)
- Sarcopenia (loss of muscle and frailty)

There are two inflammatory pathways that your system follows, which depends on the materials at hand. These materials come directly from diet and environment. All cell membranes are populated with polyunsaturated fatty acids (PUFA) that form part of the lipid bilayer in which reside working proteins, receptors, channels, and so on. The PUFAs also provide the building blocks for the inflammatory pathways. If you have cell membranes filled with omega-6 PUFAs, these become precursors for the highly inflammatory and damaging arachidonic acid pathway. Remember that many of our NSAIDs target this pathway as a way to treat inflammation. If you have cell membranes filled with more omega-3 PUFAs (EPA and DIIA), you will follow a less damaging and more healing pathway. Omega-3s can prevent the production of eicosanoids like prostaglandins and leukotrienes that normally form from the omega-6 precursors, and which are painful and damaging. While omega-6s generally become dangerous prostaglandins, omega-3s become friendly molecules. The omega-3 PUFAs also inhibit leukocyte chemotaxis, adhesion molecule expression, and the adhesive interactions of leukocytes and the endothelium. Omega-3 PUFAs allow for the production of anti-inflammatory compounds.

It's apparent that omega-3s help reduce inflammation. By reducing inflammation, noncommunicable chronic disease can be reduced or even eliminated. More omega-3s will reduce your arthritis pain.

In contrast, let's move on to omega-6s. These polyunsaturated fatty acids are found in corn oil, safflower oil, sunflower oil, grapeseed oil, soy oil, peanut oil, and vegetable oil; mayonnaise; and many salad dressings. They are also found in all grain- and corn-fed animal proteins, including most farmed fish. Some omega-6s tend to *promote*, rather than reduce, inflammation by damaging cells. Many attribute the rise of obesity, inflammation, and chronic disease to the escalation of corn and soybean oils in our processed foods.

A high level of omega-6s leads to autoimmune disorders such as rheumatoid arthritis, irritable bowel disease, type 1 diabetes, Guillain-Barre syndrome, psoriasis, celiac disease, Graves' disease, multiple sclerosis, lupus, myasthenia gravis, Addison's disease, pernicious anemia, and loss of muscle mass.[1]

If your cell membranes are filled with omega-6 fatty acids and not with omega-3s, you will only have the precursors for damaging inflammation and self-attack. Omega-6 induces that arachidonic acid pathway. Omega-3s are the building blocks needed for the repair and restoration phase. Many of today's pharmaceutical anti-inflammatory drugs target this pathway.

So, your omega-3 and omega-6 fatty acids need to be in balance. If you are a typical American, you definitely need to consume more omega-3s. There is a way to measure omega-3 levels in the bloodstream, especially the DHA and EPA levels, in the red blood cell membranes. This gives a good average of one's overall status. An omega-3 index over 8 percent is good and associated with health. Most Americans are at less than 5 percent. Most Japanese are over 10 percent, and they have a life expectancy of at least five years more than we do.[2] But the Japanese are also more active in their older years than are we; they are already incorporating this protocol!

The brain is particularly vulnerable to oxidative stress and chronic inflammation, because your brain cells need a substantial amount of glucose and oxygen. In fact, the brain consumes about 20 percent of the total amount of glucose the body needs for fuel. This means that huge amounts of mitochondria are always active in the brain and producing ATP with the byproduct of free radicals. These can lead to oxidative stress and inflammation inside the brain. Omega-3s are protective here by improving cell membranes and reducing inflammation. They make it easier to regulate emotions and have self-control and resiliency. This helps you feel better and handle stress better. Stress management is a key to enjoying less pain in life and is integral to a positive mindset for health.

FIGHTING PHRASES: OXIDATIVE STRESS AND CHRONIC INFLAMMATION

Oxidative stress and chronic inflammation are complex subjects of significant importance. Your diet, lifestyle, and environment determine whether you'll experience oxidative stress and chronic inflammation. These two threats are the source of most pain and cognitive decline, cardiovascular disease, cancers, and much of what we used to consider "aging." Most musculoskeletal pain and dysfunction are directly tied to diet and lifestyle. Arthritis is not mandatory as we age, nor are other NCDs. Many still believe that chronic diseases are due to genetics, but they are in fact a byproduct of our processed lives.

Granted, your genes provide the ammunition in your war against disease and aging. And many modern conditions and diseases—heart disease, stroke, cancer, Alzheimer's disease, osteoporosis, kidney disease, and diabetes—have some genetic link. For example, we know that carriers of two copies of the APOE-4 allele on chromosome nineteen will confer an eight-to- fifteen-fold risk of developing Alzheimer's. (That said, only 2 to 5 percent of people carry two copies of this allele.)

But you're not a victim. Genetic effects can be altered. You control your epigenetics. You serve as the commander-in-chief on your battlefield. Genes can be turned on or off depending on signals produced by the body. In fact, the vast majority of your health and how you feel is simply due to your stress, sleep quality, mindset, diet, and lifestyle. Not everything is preordained.

"HIGH ENERGY" OR "LOW ENERGY": WHICH ARE YOU AND WHY?

Do you drag yourself out of bed in the mornings? Do you feel a dip in energy right after lunch? Or maybe you experience that late-afternoon foggy feeling? That fatigue doesn't happen because you haven't yet been "caffeinated," or because you're getting sick, or because you had a little too much fun during a late night on the town.

Chalk that foggy feeling up to cellular fatigue. If the billions of cells that comprise the human body don't make enough energy to perform the daily duties of cells, then you feel fatigued overall—from head to toe.

When you eat and digest food, the electrons and energy stored in its fat, protein, and carbohydrates are harnessed by the part of your cells called mitochondria. Electrons are the Universe's way to transmit energy. They carry a charge. Food is held together by chemical bonds that hold that energy. Breaking those bonds releases the energy. The mitochondria are the real engines of your cells, refining fuel found in food by liberating its energy through a series of chemical reactions.

From that point, your organs and various systems (nervous, respiratory, digestive, musculoskeletal, and so forth) use that energy produced by your cells' mitochondria to work properly. The mitochondria produce a molecule called adenosine triphosphate (ATP), the form of energy most usable by a cell. ATP allows the movement of energy from food to where it's needed. This process is straightforward.

Briefly, when the mitochondria add a phosphate group to the molecules of adenosine monophosphate (AMP) or adenosine diphosphate (ADP), they are adding energy to the molecule. This is because the chemical bond that connects the phosphate group to the adenosine is a high-energy bond. When that bond is later broken, the energy is released and harnessed. Every single day, we turn over the equivalent of our body weight in ATP. Like gasoline or electricity formed from crude oil, ATP is the primary refined fuel used by your body, formed from basic macronutrients. The process of refining glucose and other foods into ATP produces waste products. These are called reactive oxygen species (ROS) or, more commonly, "free radicals." These are like the exhaust of engines. With oxidative phosphorylation, ATP is generated and allows for the energy of food to be released. The process requires oxygen, and the production byproducts are not just free radicals and reactive oxygen species, but also carbon dioxide and water. Therefore, we eat, breathe, and urinate.

Free radicals are a necessary part of the fuel-production process at the cellular level. But problems arise when your body produces too many free radicals, allowing landfills of waste to form in your cells, leaving your mitochondria at a very high risk for oxidative stress. This would be similar to running a car with the door closed in a garage. Eventually, the byproducts build up enough to cause harm or even death.

Reactive oxygen species tend to donate oxygen to other molecules. This is due to the complex chemistry of the outer shells of the oxygen molecule. There are electrons there that don't like to be alone. Any molecule with an unpaired electron becomes a cellular assassin, aka a free radical.

Mother Nature doesn't like an unpaired electron. These free radicals damage what they hit. They can cause molecules of other compounds in your body to disintegrate faster than a mouthful of cotton candy! And again, this disintegration causes even more oxidative stress.

OXIDATIVE STRESS PRODUCES REAL DISTRESS

Free radicals work like cluster bombs, going off everywhere in your body. They attack your DNA. They attack proteins and cell membranes in your body. Having a certain number of free radicals in your body is normal. You need a few of them because their presence tells you that you're in a period of stress. They signal other molecules and create some helpful pathways through your body.

But having too many of these free radicals creates oxidative stress, which increases inflammation that can then cause pain: diabetes pain, arthritis pain, tendinitis pain, muscle pain, bone pain. Inflammation and the over-load of free radicals also contribute to cancer, Alzheimer's, Parkinson's, and other noncommunicable chronic diseases. In fact, you can name almost any degenerative condition, and one large source of that condition is likely free radicals and/or chronic inflammation. In short, these free radicals are a byproduct of your metabolism, completely normal but hugely damaging in excess.

Most orthopedic conditions thought to be due to age or to "wear and tear" are also due to this chemical process.

When you see a rusty nail, you're seeing a type of oxidative stress. The metal becomes iron oxide—oxygen meets metal and turns it into rust.

LET'S DISCUSS ADVANCED GLYCATION END PRODUCTS

Glycation is the natural process when sugar in your bloodstream attaches to proteins or fats and forms new pro-oxidant molecules called advanced glyca-tion end products (AGEs). This process requires no enzymes and occurs spon-taneously. This means it will happen all the time, with no regulation. One of the impacts of AGEs is to inhibit normal motion and flexibility.

These AGEs—which I call monster proteins—do not just form sponta-neously inside our bodies. They can also come directly from foods we eat. These are called *dietary* advanced glycation end products, or dAGEs. Therefore, we can compound the inevitability of their formation by eating more and more of them. Ultraprocessed foods are replete with AGEs, as are most meats. Guess what foods have fewer of these monster proteins? The foods common to the Mediterranean lifestyle: whole grains, fruits, vegetables, milk, legumes, fish. These foods seem to form fewer AGEs, even with cooking. Cooking in high, dry heat enhances the formation of these damaging molecules, especially in meats. This is why I am no fan of the air fryer in my house. Fried foods are also known to increase levels of AGEs.

AGEs tend to focus on long-lived proteins, like those of your musculoskeletal system. When these AGEs move into your body's connective tissue, the makeup of that tissue changes, becoming stiff and painful. AGEs lead directly to more tissue inflammation and further oxidative stress damage.[3]

AGE deposits in connective tissue, for instance, can cause problems. In the Achilles tendon, AGEs result in thickening and stiffness. When these tissues lose elasticity, the tendon loses the ability to store energy during walking. The tendon becomes "disorganized," causing tendinitis, with the accompanying stiffness and pain. The same process occurs in cartilage. In my practice, when operating on the tendons and ligaments of people with chronic diabetes, I notice the slightly brown and dry appearance of these structures. Normal ones are shiny, white, and glistening.

Overall, AGEs can contribute to most of the aches and pains, vision loss, balance issues, nerve problems, and stiffness people typically associate with "getting older." But you can reduce all this damage by reducing AGEs in your diet, controlling glucose levels in your blood, consuming antioxidants, and moving, since skeletal muscle pulls glucose out of blood. This means avoiding ultraprocessed foods, an excessive consumption of foods derived from animals, and foods cooked with high heat, and focusing instead on the Mediterranean diet based on whole foods cooked at home. Controlling the damage caused by AGEs also depends on recruiting an army of antioxidants.

HOW YOUR ANTIOXIDANT ARMY DEFENDS YOU

If you're a football fan, you understand the concept of man-to-man defense. If the opponents have a star running back, the coach lines up (or pairs) a great linebacker to neutralize that running back's performance.

In the same way, antioxidants neutralize free radicals by donating or accepting an electron (pairing). Like a combat unit in battle, these antioxidants rush in to pair with unstable free radicals. In that pairing, they neutralize those free radicals and prevent them from harming other molecules in the body. These are so-called single-molecule antioxidants. This is a group that includes vitamin C, vitamin E, and others. There is another group of antioxidants that are enzymes. These proteins catalyze reactions that convert a molecule with an unpaired electron into one that is more stable. Part of your job is to shore up your defense capabilities by increasing the levels of both types.

So, what else can you do to "neutralize" these free radicals causing oxidative stress?

Exercise, for one thing. Although exercise temporarily increases free radicals, causing oxidative stress in your muscles, free radicals formed during exercise eventually regulate tissue growth and actually stimulate the production of more antioxidants. The mild oxidant stress of exercise causes a stress response that is beneficial. Exercise also pulls excess glucose out of the blood quickly, without the need for insulin. Reduced serum glucose means fewer AGEs, less inflammation, and less oxidative stress, and reduced activity of NF-kB, the transcription factor responsible for causing much of our inflammation.

A great way to increase antioxidants is by eating richly colored fruits and vegetables like cherries, blueberries, and green, leafy veggies. Berries are filled with potent antioxidants and may be one of your best defense sources. The Mediterranean diet pattern has high loads of antioxidants.

Nutrition Journal published a comprehensive list that rates more than three thousand foods as to their antioxidant content.[4] You can find this article online at the NIH's National Library of Medicine by searching for "the total antioxidant content of more than 3100 foods." Select from these natural antioxidants to neutralize those free radicals so they aren't creating havoc inside your body.

An easier way to try to get enough of these cellular protectors is to simply follow the Mediterranean guideline of eating between six and nine servings of vegetables and two or three servings of fruit each and every day. Too difficult? I supplement with many natural antioxidants and anti-inflammatory molecules because I find it impossible to eat that many veggies during a normal day. Supplementation is a good way to make up the balance you are missing. Another trick that works well for me is to eat muesli and add inulin or psyllium husk fiber to it. I also try to eat a lot of soups as these are a great way to sneak in many servings of vegetables.

HOW DO WE KNOW THE MEDITERRANEAN LIFESTYLE EATING PLAN WORKS SO WELL?

This lifestyle diet is better than any drug we have—better than statins, better than stents, better than steroids. Numerous studies show tremendous results from such a diet:

- Lowers rate of cardiovascular disease by 33 percent:[5] The omega-3s in the diet reduce inflammation, prevent arrhythmias, and decrease the synthesis of proinflammatory cytokines.
- Lowers risk of heart attacks by 72 percent[6]
- Reduces LDL (bad cholesterol)
- Decreases cancer incidence and mortality[7]
- Decreases overall mortality:[8] Those on a Mediterranean diet were 45 percent less likely to die than those on a low-fat diet.
- Reduces age-related cognitive decline[9]
- Lowers risk of type 2 diabetes by 19 percent[10]
- Decreases obesity[11]
- Lowers inflammation in general
- Reduces incidence of and symptoms of arthritis and other musculo-skeletal conditions.

A consistent intake of antioxidants (either through food or supplements) will counteract your body's production of free radicals and reduce oxidative stress, and chronic inflammation, and damage to your mitochondria, DNA, and cell membranes. In addition to the cleanup-and-repair tasks, this eating plan also promotes overall cell longevity.

In short, you'll live longer as you feel better now!

SO NUTRITION REALLY MATTERS?

The China Study is one of the most comprehensive nutrition studies ever carried out. It examined sixty-five counties in China, using blood tests and extensive questionnaires, gathering information on 6,500 adults.[12] Key findings include the following:

- The lower the percentage of animal protein, the greater the health benefits.
- A whole-foods, plant-based diet delivers benefits for various diseases.
- Not only can such a diet prevent disease, but it can even reverse chronic diseases like heart disease and specific cancers.
- A plant-based diet is positively linked to longevity.

The Blue Zones study is equally convincing.[13] Researchers found that the longest-living and healthiest people in the world live in these five zones: the Barbagia region of Sardinia; Ikaria, Greece; the Nicoya Peninsula, Costa Rica; Okinawa, Japan; Seventh-Day Adventists living around Loma Linda, California. (This California group lives ten years longer than their other North American counterparts.)[14]

Here's what researchers found that each of these five population groups had in common:

- They eat wisely. That includes eating their smallest meal in the late afternoon or early evening, and they don't eat for the rest of the day. Beans are the main food. They eat meat only four to five times per month. Serving sizes are three to four ounces. All but the Seventh-Day Adventists drink alcohol moderately (one to two glasses of wine per day). The Seventh-Day Adventists drink no alcohol.
- They get plenty of exercise naturally as they go about daily tasks. They don't need to train for marathons or pump iron to strengthen their muscles.
- They have a sense of purpose that gives them a positive outlook on life.
- They have routines in their daily life that help them shed stress (meditation, prayer, naps).

- They connect with others socially. All but five of the 263 centenarians interviewed belonged to some faith-based community. The researchers say attending faith-based services four times each month will add four to fourteen years to life expectancy.
- They put their loved ones before themselves. That is, they keep aging parents and grandparents nearby, which lowers disease and mortality rates of children in the home as well. Most are active in social circles that support healthy habits.

WHAT'S YOUR GUT GOT TO DO WITH IT?

Plenty—besides the obvious that what you put in your mouth affects your gut (your digestive tract). Your gut consists of more than one hundred trillion microbes (your microbiome) that are both helpful and potentially harmful. A few of these microbes are natural to our bodies; the vast majority come from the outside. For the most part, these good and bad microbes play nice with each other.

But on occasion, they can create either an inflammatory or anti-inflammatory response within your digestive tract and immune system.

The metabolic processes of good microbes (bacteria) lead to the substances that your body requires for optimal health. That is, the good bacteria in your gut help in these ways:

- How your immune system works
- How your food moves through your digestive tract
- How your body absorbs nutrients from your food and rids itself of toxins
- How your body synthesizes the molecules it requires

By contrast, the bad microbes don't produce any necessary substances in your body, and some of these microbes actually produce toxins throughout your system. What we eat either keeps these microbes in balance or out of balance. When the bad bacteria overpower the good bacteria, you'll have a negative imbalance in your microbiome.

So how does your microbiome get negatively "out of balance"? There are several ways:

- Stress
- Overusing antibiotics
- Food-borne bacteria that cause infections
- Heavy metals and pesticides from contaminated foods
- Alcohol misuse
- Diets high in processed meats, sugar, and simple carbohydrates[15]
- Low-fiber diets
- High-fructose diets

When your microbiome has more bad bacteria than good, that leads to acid reflux, food intolerance, diabetes,[16] skin concerns, mood disorders, chronic fatigue, inflammation of your nerves, dementia, and other digestive problems.

Poor diets can also affect your microbiome by causing the lining of your intestines to become permeable (known as "leaky gut"). Microbes leaking from your gut into the bloodstream can generate chronic inflammation, lead to a tumor, cause an autoimmune response, or even increase the size of blockages in your arteries. Gut microbes can send signals to your central nervous system, which in turn affects your physical brain function and emotional behaviors.

In summary, your microbiome directly affects how you digest food, how susceptible you are to diseases, and your overall health.

As you've read through this technical explanation of what happens to food inside your body as it turns into energy, you may have come to a startling realization: Harmful foods cause oxidative stress, chronic inflammation, and AGE formation. Chronic overload of these metabolic dysfunctions leads to various diseases and conditions.[17] So we're back to the critical importance of what you put in your mouth to metabolize. Quality food leads to a longer, healthier life. A quality diet, combined with a good schedule, mindset, and exercise can dramatically change how your body functions and feels. Know that there will never be a double-blind, placebo-controlled study of a healthy life. But also know there are few, if any, side effects of leading a clean and healthy life. In addition, all the data we have to date seems to indicate that the combination of MEDS will give you that healthy life and you will feel much better.

Now that we've talked about how we get sick and the importance of lifestyle, let's take a look at the first part of the MEDS protocol: mindset.

Chapter Three

THE RADICAL POWER OF A POSITIVE MINDSET

Every negative belief weakens the partnership between mind and body.

—Deepak Chopra

Warning: You're about to enter a stress-free zone of positive thoughts and inspirational messages (as you can tell from the quotation above). But don't jump to the wrong conclusion that this has nothing to do with scientific theories and evidence. You'll find plenty of studies supporting the mind-body connection. Move ahead at your own discretion.

The premise of my protocol is that aches, pains, stiffness, soreness, and other body problems you have can be avoided, managed, and potentially reversed with MEDS—mindset, exercise, diet, sleep. Each aspect of the protocol links to the others, and they self-reinforce and synergize. In order for you to move forward on this journey and create the brain and body you want, a health mindset is mandatory.

A health mindset will allow you to feel less pain and respond better to stress. You will have greater mental and physical resiliency. A health mindset will give you self-control and the ability to resist temptations that will keep you from your goal of a strong and healthy body and brain. A health mindset provides insight that helps you make better decisions about your health.

What is a mindset? According to the Oxford English Dictionary, the definition of mindset is "the established set of attitudes." The medical definition is more nuanced: core assumptions held about domains or categories of things that orient us to a particular set of expectations, explanations, and goals. Mindsets are a way of viewing reality and will shape what we understand, what we expect, and what we do and feel. Studies show that a positive mindset has profound benefits for the neuroendocrine and immune systems,[1] and can also modify an individual's experience of pain.[2] Reducing stress, being around happy people, strengthening your social relationships, eating brain foods, and sleeping all help with positive moods. If you think you are negative, please understand you can become positive. Once you gain the health mindset, change is inevitable.

MINDSET AND PAIN

As an orthopedic surgeon serving in the conflicts in both Iraq and Afghanistan, I've witnessed firsthand the importance of a positive mindset. I still recall a fragile but fervently pleading soldier who was a patient in our base hospital. Only a few weeks after he'd had both legs blown off by an IED, he begged me to clear him to return to the field with his team. He was in no shape physically to return to the battlefield. But mentally in shape? A morale-building mindset if I ever met one! He later went on to obtain prostheses and continued to serve our country with honor. The work done at the Center for the Intrepid at Brooke Army Medical Center is a testament to both science and the power of mindset.

There is a distinct difference between impairment and disability. You can be impaired without being disabled. Mindset plays a fundamental role in all aspects of orthopedic medicine. A few decades ago in the chronic-pain world, the biopsychosocial aspects of care became abundantly clear. Only in the past few years has the orthopedic world started to catch on. I am going to teach you—once again—how much of what you feel and do is totally in your control.

I want you to understand that you do not need to turn over control of your life, your abilities, and how you feel to doctors, drugs, and dysfunctional hospitals.

UNDERSTANDING MINDSET IN THE CLINICAL SETTING

I was taught that good surgeons had good outcomes and bad surgeons did not. However, this never reconciled how surgeons with a good bedside manner, even when lacking in technical skill, seemed to always have happy patients and good outcomes. Now, after years of research and experience, I understand that a good bedside manner is code for a deep, intrinsic understanding of mindset. Really good surgeons should be technically great, but they also need to positively direct the patient's mindset. At this point, you may be asking, "Are you saying that how we feel mentally and emotionally affects whether our surgery corrects a problem?" Yes. That's exactly what I am saying and what scientific studies prove.

In a study conducted at Yale University, three physician researchers reviewed and analyzed twenty-nine published reports regarding psychological factors related to surgery outcomes. The studies included varied types of surgery, and the researcher used five clinical criteria to measure surgical outcomes. These criteria were pain levels, procedure factors, length of hospital stay, functional recovery, and physical recovery as reported by the patient and documented clinically. Functional recovery is important, as this indicates the patient is perhaps working again, but at least able to do daily tasks of living such as cooking, cleaning, going to church. If a patient simply sits on a couch all day, this is not considered a good functional result.

As far as the psychological factors they measured against, the researchers looked at the patients' anxiety, stress, worry, anger/hostility, depression, general emotional state, moods, and attitudes. For example, what were their perceptions and beliefs about the control they felt they had over their lives? Were they generally optimistic or pessimistic? Did they have positive or negative expectations about the surgery? What was their ability to cope with real pain? What personality characteristics did they exhibit, such as neuroticism, extroversion, sense of self-esteem, motivation, ego strength, feelings of inadequacy?

These twenty-nine controlled studies revealed that all of these psychosocial characteristics did in fact closely predict surgical outcomes, both positive and negative. In particular, a patient's mood and attitude influenced their surgery outcome, including their need for pain medicine, the length of their hospital stay, how quickly they could return to normal function, and even patient self-ratings on their recovery, more than any clinical factor. This means mindset mattered the most for the clinical results.[3]

Orthopedic-specific studies report similar findings about how negative emotions, depression, personality traits, and long-held beliefs are closely related to the current pain the patients feel.[4] Something as simple as the diagnostic label will make patients without a health mindset feel more hopeless and helpless than those with more optimism. For example, pessimistic, depressed patients believe that pain indicates damage and that their pain is never going to get better.

In orthopedic surgery, your mindset is critical. This means that you are in total control of how you feel, both after surgery and before surgery. For orthopedic surgeons, it is becoming quite clear that functional outcomes depend upon the patient's coping skills, social support, and levels of anxiety and depression. Note that I did not say anything about the diagnosis or technical aspects of surgery. Evidence proves that your emotional health matters the most when it comes to the outcomes of orthopedic surgeries.[5]

Every year we learn more about how outcomes in orthopedics have more to do with patient factors than surgery-related factors. Regarding the spine, good emotional health before surgery is predictive of better results, while low emotional health is predictive of poor outcomes.[6] For the hip, poor emotional health along with depression and another site of osteoarthritis predicts an unsatisfied patient up to a year after surgery.[7] Finally, for the knee, even if your postoperative films look amazing, if you had poor emotional health before surgery, you are far less likely to improve physically afterward.[8]

How can outcomes be related to the emotional health of a patient? The key is found in complex interconnections between body and brain. There is a wonderful study from 2007 by Alia Crum that shows the control the brain has over your body. The authors took two groups of hotel room attendants. Both groups were taught the massive importance of daily exercise for health. One group was educated as to how their normal work activities satisfied recommendations for healthy daily exercise. The other group did not receive this teaching. Each group was measured for blood pressure, body fat, waist-to-hip ratio, and weight/BMI before and after the four-week study. Guess what happened? Those who learned that their daily activities were healthy and beneficial improved in all the health parameters measured. The other group did not. In neither group did any of their activities change at all during the study. The only thing that changed was the mindset of that one group.[9] This means that just the knowledge and belief that something is healthy can change internal physiology. This is amazing, I think.

PLACEBOS AND THE MIND-BODY CONNECTION

The best science-based evidence of the mind-body connection are placebos in clinical trials, which we've discussed earlier in the book. When patients are given fake treatments so that researchers can compare their results with patient outcomes of those who've received a real treatment, many in the placebo group report they feel better. You'll recall that placebos such as bloodletting, sugar pills, bread pills, and mild ointments have been used for centuries in the treatment of pain—often with favorable outcomes. That is, patients report feeling better even when their "treatment" should have absolutely no impact on their condition or illness.

The word *mesmerize* originated from the work of Dr. Franz Mesmer in the eighteenth century. He created the technique of "animal magnetism" to treat many patients across Europe, involving an elaborate performance for the patient that caused them to be "cured." Other physicians suspected this was a placebo. Mesmer was eventually discredited by Benjamin Franklin, who developed the double-blind trial to disprove Mesmer's techniques.[10]

Don't be *mesmerized* by your MRI results or by a surgeon telling you surgery is the only answer. Don't be mesmerized when your doctors says you will always be in pain and stiffness is inevitable after the age of forty.

Placebos work through the endogenous opioid and cannabinoid pathways. When people are given naloxone, an opioid blocker, placebo effects fail. Expectations can cause the release of your self-made opioids and other pain-relieving molecules, a process proven with neuroimaging studies and biomarkers. For a placebo to trigger this release, you must *believe* that the placebo will work. This means all the power of that molecular connection resides in your brain. If you don't believe that a particular treatment will work, your brain will instead trigger the release of molecules (cholecystokinin) that increase anxiety, pain, and hyperalgesia (excessive pain).[11] If you are convinced that you are doomed, then you will be doomed.

You too may have used your mind-over-matter strength on occasion, as most of us have at one time or another. You've had the flu and felt lousy, but you put aside your pain to care for another sick family member. Moms of young children force themselves to do this routinely. Or you feel a little sick or fatigued, but you really want to attend a big event, so you pull yourself together and go. While at the party, you amazingly forget about your pain. But soon after returning home, you soon feel sick again. Even patients with debilitating pain report distracting themselves with a funny movie or an intriguing novel. There is a lot of research happening with virtual reality utilizing the technique of distraction to reduce pain. Distraction is simply an element of attention, and part of a health mindset is to change your attention.

Surgery has, on occasion, been called the ultimate placebo.[12] The data from sham surgery studies has proven this to be true. For example, in a study of subjects five years after sham or real meniscal surgery, the meniscectomy group (real surgery) did not have better results than the fake surgery group. In contrast, the real surgery group had more arthritis than the fake surgery group.[13] It is clear that, for some patients, surgery is not superior to either fake surgery or physical therapy.[14] Despite this knowledge, more surgery is done now than ever before. Obviously, most surgeons do not wish to believe this information.

One argument against the data of sham surgery studies in orthopedics is that some of them come out of Finland and Denmark. It is said that the Finns have *sisu*, which is a type of determination, grit, and courage. The Danes are said to have *hygge*, which denotes gratitude, appreciation, and happiness. These mindsets are said to account for the results of placebo-controlled surgeries.[15] To me, this is not a disparagement of the data from multiple sham-surgery studies, but rather a testament to the power of mindset. I just hope that they don't mean that the rest of us lack such grit, gratitude, happiness, and courage and will never be good enough to avoid surgery.

It is not just surgery that should be avoided. I am an advocate for avoiding steroid shots if possible. For one thing, insurance companies take full advantage of the status quo bias to manipulate many doctors into believing steroids are a good thing.[16] They are just cheap, not necessarily good. Evidence clearly proves placebo injections are safer and have good results when compared to steroids. Evidence also shows that steroids can damage musculoskeletal tissues over time.[17] Think about this: steroid injection and knee arthroscopy rates are increasing despite the studies proving they advance arthritis. Meanwhile, total joint replacement rates are also increasing. If steroid injections and knee scopes were so great, why are more and more people developing arthritis? Every middle-aged person who walks into a doctor's office with knee pain today can expect multiple injections, a scope or two or three, and then a replacement. While this is standard and acceptable to most, I am offering you a way to exit this treadmill. The status quo is steroids and surgery, and nobody wants to be the first to change. I want things to change for the better and to give the power of how your body feels back to you and your mind.

You need to avoid a pain mindset. You can do this because your brain has the ability to modify its perception of the electrical signals that it receives. One of the main ways the brain does this is via descending inhibition pathways. There is abundant crosstalk between your brain and body. This is both chemical and electrical. The brain and nervous system are also plastic—that is, they are able to change. Pain is meant to be merely a danger signal to the brain. When a certain stimulus happens (heat, cold, cut, contusion, etc.), the receptors at that spot will send a signal to the brain that will be interpreted as pain. This is useful to then allow us to get away from whatever the problem is. This becomes problematic if there is no actual danger and no real reason to have that signal. Pain is not the same as nociception. It is fully subjective. Any given signal will be amplified or dampened by the brain depending on certain variables, the health of the brain, prior training or conditioning, and any neuroinflammation.

Descending inhibition is the top-down control of pain. The electrical signal that moves from the receptor, up the spinal cord, into various parts of the brain, and back down again are totally modifiable. Variables that are able to act on the brain to modify perceived pain include emotions, environment, mood, memory, expectations, experience, attention. The brain will take all variables into account and produce a perception for you. That perception can be intense pain or not. In other words, by way of the descending inhibitory pathways, you have the power to either facilitate or inhibit any given stimulus. All of this can be trained and changed as desired.

You can use techniques to manipulate your mood and your expectations, and to change your attention and modify these pathways to lessen the perception of pain.[18] When pain stops serving its given purpose of protection and becomes its own sort of disease, this ability is necessary.

By harnessing the power of the inhibitory pathways against pain, you can avoid what is called central sensitization. This is a situation seen in many with chronic pain. With central sensitization, pain is amplified and widespread pain becomes common. If you are unable to have a healthy mindset, then you experience the nocebo effect, where there is an expectation of pain or treatment failure and all of the internal pain inhibition systems are turned off. The nocebo effect is the opposite of the placebo effect. Sadly, it is just as powerful.

Mindfulness is one way to harness the power of your descending inhibitory pathways to control pain and stress. This is a tool that allows you to gain a more positive mindset. Mindfulness-based modification of pain works, and this has been proven by chronic pain science. Mindfulness can help reduce pain in fibromyalgia, rheumatoid arthritis, migraines, irritable bowel syndrome, orthopedic conditions, and many more. Mindfulness is thought to be especially good at reducing what are known as the affective components of pain. These are the emotional and mental aspects that accompany pain and make it worse. These include a lack of pain acceptance, depression, catastrophizing, and stress.

Mindfulness training increases activation of certain areas in your brain important for pain perception.

Basically, your brain can recategorize pain as just another type of sensory information. If you get good at this, what used to be felt as noxious pain suddenly becomes merely annoying. What you must develop is a superior sense of pain acceptance with a belief that you can handle it. Once you achieve that, your brain will do the rest of the work for you.

Being a veteran, I always think of the military's saying, "Pain is weakness leaving the body." Though it seems trite, this saying is a strong method for enhancing mindsets to improve performance and decrease perceived pain.

A calm mind brings inner strength and self-confidence, so that's very important for good health.
—DALAI LAMA, HEAD OF STATE IN TIBET

When someone feels pain, they often second-guess themselves, wondering how much of their pain is real and how much might be caused by their state of mind. Many others believe that pain must mean that something is wrong or broken. This is not always true. Think of the confusion after a family member, Josh, a seventy-five-year-old male, had been diagnosed with prostate cancer. After his oncologist had given up on radiation treatments when the cancer spread to his bones, Josh reported severe back pain. As he lay in bed with a morphine pump in his back, he asked these questions of his caretakers:

"Is the cancer causing my back pain?"
"Does my back hurt so bad because I'm depressed?"
"Does my back hurt from lying here all day?"

Of course, his family had no way of knowing the extent of his pain or how his mindset affected the pain he endured. Eventually, Josh himself decided that his depression was the culprit and asked to have the morphine pump removed from his back. The lack of morphine did not affect the pain he felt, and in time, the pain resolved. It was simply due to the depression and lack of activity during his treatments. John became aware of this and changed his mindset without any help.

I tell you about Josh only to say that maybe you too have similar concerns and questions. Some pain you feel may be related to physical causes, and some may be a result of your mindset. Step one of gaining a healthy mindset is to create awareness of your current thoughts.

When physicians assure their patients that their pain comes from physical causes and fail to understand the mind-body connection, they still determine to put mind over matter, so to speak. By coaching a patient that there is an anatomic source of the pain, that pain is then always attached to that source. This then becomes an anchoring bias for the patient. I see this all the time in my clinic. For instance, patients present to me after the failure of treatments elsewhere to address their back pain. Despite the lack of success with therapeutics all designed for "discogenic" pain, these patients often hold on very tightly to the belief that a disc is the source of their pain. After all, a doctor or two before me told them it was on the MRI. The bias was reinforced with repetition by the doctors.

NOCEBO AND MIND CONTROL

To more fully understand the placebo effect, it will help to understand some of the main factors that drive the nocebo effect—that is, the factors that make pain worse for you. Scientists know that cognition, emotions, expectations, cultural beliefs about pain, childhood experiences, and stress levels can influence pain. But one of the most important factors in terms of pain control is your level of pain catastrophizing. A person's response to any given arthritic joint, stiff and painful tendon, and muscle tear is heavily influenced by their memories, priming, and conditioning. It is entirely possible to reduce pain simply by believing that you can. Likewise, pain can be made much worse simply by not believing that you can manage it, and that it will worsen. This is the difference between placebo and nocebo—and you can control it. Nocebo is largely influenced by your personal level of pain catastrophizing. The nocebo effect is a large reason why costs rise while treatment success falls.

Pain catastrophizing is a persistent pattern of distressing emotion and thought processes related to current or even anticipated pain. This situation involves ruminations on pain, feelings of helplessness about pain, and the consequent magnification of that pain.[19] People who catastrophize will have more pain, use more opioids, stay in hospitals longer, have delayed recovery, and have poor outcomes from surgery. In fact, it is one of the strongest predictors of pain treatment outcomes.[20] People who think of pain in catastrophic ways have loss of mass in areas of the brain that are key for the descending modulation of pain signals. Their brains become primed for pain.

The medical and pharmaceutical industries have trained us to believe that using our own minds to modify our pain experience is only worth trying if everything else they offer has failed. This is false. The truth of the matter is that they have used the placebo and nocebo against us for years. The opioid epidemic is a great example of that.

I was taught that pain is the "fifth vital sign" and that the goal of any treatment is a zero on the pain scale. This has created the expectation that any pain is bad pain, and that any treatment that does not achieve a zero on the scale is a failure. This particular mindset has created a nation filled with addicts and increasing numbers of people believing themselves to be disabled. The industry created the belief that narcotics would eliminate pain, increase function, and solve a person's problems without addiction (placebo) and, at the same time, convinced people that stopping narcotics would be painful and create horrible withdrawal symptoms (nocebo).

Many of my patients have come to me looking for natural solutions for their pain. They do not want to be on narcotics. However, when they asked their pain-management physicians about stopping, they were told that their pain would return, there was no cure for their condition, and the only possible answer was narcotic therapy. In addition, anytime opioids lose efficacy—as they always do because of physical tolerance—to avoid the potential for withdrawal, most pain physicians would escalate dosing rather than work on a taper with patients. They harnessed negative beliefs about stopping narcotics to increase the need for the ongoing, monthly prescriptions.

A wonderful study demonstrates the power of the mind in terms of pain control. In this study, there were three groups, and each group received IV remifentanil after a heat-pain stimulus. One group was told they were receiving a very powerful painkiller. The second group was told they were receiving saline and would continue to have some pain. The third group was told they were receiving an agent that would increase their pain. So, the first group was expecting something positive, the second group was expecting a neutral situation, and the third group was expecting the worst. The results were amazing. The first group had double the pain relief of the second group. The third group had no pain relief whatsoever. Remember: each group received the exact same amount of IV remifentanil.[21] Better yet, the authors showed brain neuroimaging findings consistent with changes in descending inhibition signaling.

What I want you to understand is that you are in control of your situation. Sure, you may have arthritis, you may be older, you may have stiff and creaky joints, or you may have tendinitis or a tear. What you should not have is learned helplessness. Learn techniques to enhance your brain pathways that inhibit pain.

STRESS, CORTISOL, AND PAIN

Stress causes your body to release the hormone cortisol. This fight-or-flight hormone controls inflammation, metabolism, and sleep-wake cycles. Cortisol is also a source for increased pain. Normally, cortisol is supposed to be higher in the mornings and lower in the evenings. Stress can change that healthy oscillation and keep it elevated all day and night.

Some symptoms of high cortisol levels include high blood pressure, high blood sugar, muscle weakness, weight gain, acne, thinning skin, fatigue, irritability, pain, and headaches. Controlling your stress, and therefore your cortisol levels, will make your life much better.

In a study that looked at two groups of people with or at risk for knee osteoarthritis aged forty-five to eighty-five, levels of reported pain were compared against sociodemographic factors, psychosocial stress, and levels of salivary cortisol throughout the day. The authors discovered that financial stress was a major cause of elevated cortisol in the evenings and throughout the day, and consequently also more pain.[22] I see this a lot when treating my patients at the main safety-net hospital in New Orleans. Stressful lives combined with a lack of optimism, learned helplessness, and underdeveloped coping skills lead directly to worse health outcomes and more complaints of pain. Adverse life events cause higher levels of cortisol and the development of chronic pain.[23] When you have high levels of cortisol due to stress, you will feel uneasy or a sense of impending doom. There will be rumination, worry, and fear-avoidance behaviors. Active coping and optimism are associated with less pain because of this relationship.[24] Because cortisol is so integral to inflammation, this makes sense.

I have seen many patients who think of pain in a way that guarantees they will always have it. They think about pain in a catastrophic way and allow it, or the thought of it, to control their lives. Pain catastrophizing is one way to ensure chronic stress and cortisol dysregulation. The maladaptive responses of magnification, rumination, and helplessness lead to ongoing cortisol release.[25] Eventually, these people enter a situation like a diabetic with insulin resistance. The cortisol receptors will no longer respond to the cortisol molecule, and the hormonal balance will be altered. By having exaggerated responses to stress/pain, they have constant cortisol spikes. These cause the brain to consolidate fear-based memories and responses along with cortisol spikes. This of course will make the pain worse and slow down any possible recovery.

The way to address these problems is through mindset training. Interventions of this nature are so successful in making you healthier, less stressed, and having less pain because they harness the executive control of a part of the brain known as the prefrontal cortex. Faulty and maladaptive beliefs are identified, assessed, and addressed in a proper positive fashion. Chronic stress is managed, the descending inhibition is improved for pain, and the circadian rhythm—disrupted by elevated cortisol—can return.

By changing your mindset from a pain mindset/fixed mindset to a health mindset/growth mindset, and engaging in optimism and not pessimism, you will feel better regardless of a given condition. There has never been a study that demonstrates a direct link between the level of arthritis on an X-ray and the level of pain a patient reports. This means, by definition, that pain varies despite how good or bad the X-ray appears. The initial signal for pain comes from a nociceptor, but it is heavily modified by many factors prior to being interpreted by the brain. The brain can either amplify that signal or dampen it. The choice can be placed in your hands, but to harness these powers, you must train your prefrontal cortex. This will, in turn, give you the elusive self-control necessary to achieve all of your health and life goals.

To follow my own advice about a relaxed mindset, I've focused on the positive in the rest of the chapter: how to turn off these negative triggers that harm your health and turn on peace of mind. We'll start with the easier actions first:

---

*If you don't like something, change it. If you
can't change it, change your attitude.*
—MAYA ANGELOU, AMERICAN MEMOIRIST

TRANSFORMING YOUR MIND TO TAMP DOWN YOUR PAIN

Pain is real. But you can learn ways to cope with it so that it doesn't destroy your peace of mind and your enjoyment in life. This health mindset gives you the power to fully engage the MEDS protocol.

One popular way to improve your mindset about pain is to engage in cognitive behavioral therapy for chronic pain (pCBT). This works by reducing catastrophizing and increasing self-efficacy; you are able to believe you can live with pain and manage it. During the process, you learn about the immense power of your brain and mindset in terms of the pain you feel for any given condition. You learn that you are the master of your pain, not the other way around. With pCBT, you will learn all of your personal maladaptive thoughts about pain and the neural pathways that take those thoughts and use them to amplify pain signals. Some such thoughts might be *This is never going to get better and no doctor understands me*, or *There is nothing I can do because of this pain*, or *I am at the mercy of my pain*.

With pCBT, you will learn how to calm your nervous system. You will learn to become aware of negative thoughts and how to counteract those thoughts in real time. You will learn positive distraction techniques. When you do this, you will have less pain and better function.[26] Best of all, there is no medication, and consequently, there are no side effects. One issue with pCBT is that it subscribes to the concept that pain is the same as nociception. That is, the theory holds that there is either a biomedical source or a central source (i.e., in the brain or spinal cord) for the initial pain signal and that it is the same as "pain." It is not. Pain is simply an interpretation of electricity by the brain that is designed to denote a danger signal and to stimulate protection. Pain happens with or without tissue damage, and tissue damage can happen with or without pain.

If you can't find a pCBT practitioner, or your insurance won't cover it, there are other methods you can use to enhance the health mindset. Engaging the prefrontal cortex leads to self-control, a necessary precondition for the awareness, attention, and assessment you must possess to change your mind. (Incidentally, self-control is also necessary to fight the scourge of ultraprocessed food [UPF] addiction, since additives in that food stimulate the reward/motivation sections of the brain. The properties that give such pleasure and reward eventually diminish the abilities of the prefrontal cortex and self-control becomes more difficult.)[27]

My protocol for you works best together. Each step is synergistic with the others. For example, a positive health mindset makes nutrition easier to achieve and exercise more desirable. Meanwhile, good nutrition makes achieving brain health and allowing for the neuroplasticity necessary to change to a positive mindset.

DO A DIGITAL DETOX

Social technologies fundamentally sabotage our ability to gain a health mindset in a few ways. There are actual deficits of neurotransmitters produced, there is a paradigm of false comparisons, and there is the inability to use the tool of mindfulness. If you are glued to a phone seeking reward from pictures, videos, shopping, clickbait, and so on, then you obviously cannot be present in your body in that moment.

Have you noticed that people rarely, if ever, post on Facebook, Instagram, or LinkedIn about getting jilted or going broke. Instead, their posts feature the high points in life: glamorous vacations, weddings, graduation ceremonies, fun parties with friends, career honors, and so forth. If you spend too much time on these social media platforms, it's only natural to think that everyone but you is living a glamorous life every day. They aren't. To avoid depression after comparing your daily life to the ups in everyone else's life, stay off the platform(s) for a week or month. You'll be amazed at how your stress lessens and emotions lighten up.

There is also a growing body of evidence that proves the small screens diminish levels of dopamine and other catecholamines in the brain. They trigger neural pathways that constantly demand reward and limit neural pathways that promote happiness and self-efficacy. Smartphones also increase levels of anxiety and depression and inhibit real social interactions, while overuse (especially in the evening) leads to poor sleep quality.

If you are addicted to sugar and processed foods and also constantly use smartphones, it will be difficult to follow my protocol. You will need to take things slowly to allow your brain to rewire. If you are like many Americans, you are addicted not only to sugar but also to scrolling. It is important to stop consuming excessive added sugars and processed foods. This is because sugar will change your brain in very similar ways to illicit drugs or gambling. Smartphone social and gaming apps are designed to hijack the wiring of the brain's need to seek reward as well. The combination of forced reward seeking by processed foods with added sugars and that of brilliantly engineered smartphones is amazingly powerful in controlling your brain. Change is possible, but it will require time and a bit of effort.

I do not recommend cold turkey on any of these. You have undergone a process called long-term potentiation in your brain. That is, your brain has reinforced reward pathways associated with the consumption of sugar and processed foods, together with screen scrolling. The connections in the brain have strengthened over time because of repetition of stimuli. You will need to slowly decrease the number of repeats if you want to disconnect dopamine and reward from sugar, processed foods, and smartphone apps successfully. Once you do this, simple things like a walk outside, sharing a home-cooked meal with family or friends, attending church, or reading a book will become much more pleasurable.

Almost everything will work again if you unplug
it for a few minutes, including you.
—ANNE LAMOTT, WRITER

MEDITATE TO RELIEVE STRESS

In addition to elevating cortisol levels, high stress can also deplete your adrenal glands. When your body constantly sends messages to these glands begging for more adrenaline to meet the demands of stress, soon all the systems throughout your body are working against each other to meet unrealistic calls to keep up. At some point, you may start to feel nauseated, foggy, fatigued, and totally out of control. Hormones play a major part in how we handle stress, how we process foods and fat in our body, how we sleep—and even how we handle temptation at the grocery store.

Meditation is a good way to stop all this chaos. Do keep in mind that there's not just one form of mediation. With guided meditation or visualization, for instance, someone leads you to concentrate on as many restful mental scenes as possible, encouraging you to focus on sights, sounds, smells, and textures of the visualized images.

Others learn meditation through yoga sessions, where you strike different poses as you breathe deeply to relax. And yoga has other benefits besides a positive mindset. Yoga exercises increase your flexibility and give you a better range of motion. Yoga emphasizes a balance between opposing muscle and fascial groups in the body. This is important as many orthopedic pains can be traced to simple mechanical dysfunctions that can be remedied without surgery if identified. With yoga, you also increase your muscle strength and bone density. The breathing techniques learned in yoga are especially beneficial.

Others practice meditation techniques such as Qigong, Tai Chi, or transcendental meditation (repeating a key mantra, word, or phrase to block out distracting thoughts). Prayer can also offer a very powerful method of changing your focus. Prayer can enhance gratitude, which is associated with positive and optimistic mindsets.

We feel out of sorts when we have unmet expectations and experience deep disappointments. For example, you expect weekly visits from your children or grandchildren, but they rarely show up. Or maybe you expect your spouse to run family errands, but he or she never volunteers. Or maybe you've been passed over for a big promotion and feel angry at those you consider more financially successful than you are.

Whatever your unmet expectations, you will experience disappointment until you latch onto a new perspective about issues that trouble you. Here's what one colleague told us about his newfound peace: "For months, I've felt angry at my boss because I didn't get the size bonus I had expected for successfully completing a big project. But then I started attending a book club that meets during a brown-bag lunch at work, and the topic of gratefulness came up in our discussion. It really changed my thinking. It hit me: After all, my boss didn't have to give me *any* bonus. He just did it. It's an extra $1,000 that they didn't have to hand out. I guess you could say I've gone from hateful to grateful."

Looking at the big picture with gratitude rather than expectations gives you a more positive outlook on your life.

Progressive relaxation is a useful tool when your body is going into a fight-or-flight response inappropriately. This can happen when frustrated, angry, envious, or when having pain. The most common technique in the United States, which was invented by Dr. Edmund Jacobson in the 1920s as a way to help his patients deal with anxiety, uses alternating relaxing and tensioning of muscle groups. Normally, this would be done lying down with eyes closed, but this position is not mandatory. This can even be performed when waiting in a TSA line at the airport. The technique uses opposing muscle groups. If the hamstring should relax, you would contract the quadriceps first. This harnesses the power of reciprocal relaxation and is part of yoga's success.

Jacobson's technique works on the theory that contraction of a group of muscles will cause increased relaxation of that group. You could begin with the toes and fingers and work the way to your core with this method. Just two sessions of progressive relaxation can give you results. Both styles utilize diaphragmatic breathing techniques as well.

Relaxation techniques like this put you back in control of how you might respond to pain, stress, and frustration. It helps to break the pain-muscle-tension-anxiety cycle.

Never be in a hurry; do everything quietly and in a calm spirit. Do not lose your inner peace for anything whatsoever, even if your whole world seems upset.
—ST. FRANCIS DE SALES

If most CEOs of Fortune 500 companies, celebrities, scientists, and athletes use the powers of mindset to improve their lives and performance, why wouldn't you?

The health-care and food systems have a vested interest to keep the population in a fixed or negative mindset, especially when it comes to their health, bodies, and pain. By anchoring individuals to the bias that there are biomedical reasons for their problems that can be "fixed," they force you to miss a true opportunity to elevate yourself and your family above all of the nonsense. If you gain positivity and optimism, your central control systems will downregulate any given pain signal. By becoming aware of catastrophic thoughts about pain and tissue damage, you can reappraise, assess, and modify those thoughts into more realistic ones that will actually help and not hurt. By changing your food intake and sleeping better, you can assist your brain's neuroplasticity efforts. By enhancing your own sense of self-control, you will overcome food and sugar addiction, engage more socially, have even better brain control over your body, and rise to new levels in life. A health mindset gives you the knowledge and power to make the right decisions. Mindset is everything, and you need to understand this.

In the medical world, health means there is an absence of disease. You and I want much more for ourselves. For us, health means physical health; safety; social and emotional connections; spiritual wellness; personal sense of well-being; financial health; and feeling great. All of this is achievable once you gain the health mindset.

When the brain is inflamed, depleted of neurotransmitters, and poorly wired, it is not working well for us. The critical pathways needed to improve our health and how we feel are not there. For example, pain catastrophizing causes kinesiophobia, or the fear of movement. This fear-avoidance mentality leads to brain changes that cause dysfunction and chronic pain, resulting in a state of learned helplessness.

The mechanism for this negative mindset is related to the levels and function of certain neurotransmitters in the brain, especially the dorsal raphe nucleus. Serotonin is certainly linked to learned helplessness. Interestingly, exercise can help to reverse the imbalance.

Again, the Well Theory Protocol requires eventual adoption of all steps as they each help the other.

The godfather of optimism, the late Martin Seligman, a Harvard professor, described optimism as a more internal locus of control with better self-actualization and self-efficacy. Optimists explain events in a constructive manner, they develop positive internal dialogues, and generally engage in a growth mindset.

Most of our health problems can be managed by this simple technique of increasing our own agency. Recall that descending inhibition is the top-down dampening of any unpleasant sensation like pain. Negative thoughts increase levels of pain. And expectations shape pain. They also shape your success at health. Expectations create the framework of your mind.

Chapter Four

CONSIDER EXERCISE YOUR FRIEND, NOT YOUR ENEMY

If you don't make time for exercise, you'll probably have to make time for illness.

—Robin Sharma, Canadian author

Your body is capable of so much more than you realize, and it can be your friend and not your enemy; your body can heal just about anything if given the chance. The biomechanics of its connective tissues allow your body to handle even intensive stress and strain.

The human body possesses significant mechanical complexity. You are a marvel of tension, force, compression, movement, and more. You are a marvelous design, down to the smallest organelle in your cells! Even better, your system is flexible and can adapt to changing environments and has self-repair capacity. Symmorphosis tells us that form follows function in terms of the human body.[1] I believe this to be true, inclusive of the self-repair, self-control, and self-determination abilities. When we fall apart, it is often from a lack of activity—not necessarily aging.[2] As form follows function, if you cease to function, your form (body/brain) will follow. We don't degenerate because we age. Rather, we age because we degenerate. We all know that a body in motion stays in motion, and your body is no different.

Do not think I am telling you to exercise to lose weight. The best way to lose weight is to limit the carbon buildup by limiting the intake of carbon atoms. That means portion control. It is, in fact, much easier to practice portion control than to exercise. For sure, it takes self-control to resist temptation! But think of the trick your mind plays when it convinces you that walking four miles so you can eat ice cream is easier than not eating ice cream in the first place. Most would try to do the exercise so they could get the dopamine hit, as opposed to avoiding the processed food. This does not compute.

Exercise is a legal elixir. It can reduce the following:

- Your risk of cardiovascular disease by 10–20 percent for women and 20–30 percent for men[3]
- Your risk of type 2 diabetes by 58 percent[4]
- Osteoarthritis joint and muscle pain—exercise is *the* most effective, nondrug treatment.[5] Exercise can also eliminate or reverse your risk of joint replacement.
- Your risk for dementia by 30 percent[6]
- The risk of Alzheimer's by 45 percent[7]
- Your risk of thirteen types of cancer by 12–21 percent[8]
- Your overall risk of premature death by 27 percent[9]

For any given condition, there is really no better treatment or prevention than exercise. Why this is not put forth by the massive machine that is health care in our country, I will leave for you to determine. My job with this book is to simply help you feel better and avoid surgery and other potentially harmful "treatments." So, I don't want you to exercise to lose weight. I want you to exercise to have less pain, better joints, connective tissues, and brains. If you want normal connective tissue and joints, without disease, then you must exercise. Physical inactivity begets weakness, instability, pain, imbalances, and deterioration.

IT'S NOT WEAR AND TEAR

Obviously, the concept of wear and tear is exaggerated. The population is much less active now than ever before. Despite the fact that we hardly move at all, we experience more problems with musculoskeletal disorders and disability than in the past. There is more pain. There are more NCDs. Evaluations of skeletons of those fifty years old and up from prehistory until recently demonstrate that osteoarthritis is twice as common now as it was before World War II, even accounting for increased life expectancy.[10] Paralyzed individuals have thinner cartilage than normal controls,[11] while those who exercise have thicker cartilage.[12] Clearly, overuse of the body cannot be the reason for problems like osteoarthritis. Something else is afoot.

Osteoarthritis and other musculoskeletal disorders are essentially due to metabolic syndrome, dietary changes, and physical inactivity.[13] Metabolic syndrome is a group of factors that together link to metabolic dysfunction and insulin resistance. Having this increases your risk of poor health. You must have three of the following five features to have this syndrome. Waist circumference greater than thirty-five inches for women and forty inches for men; high blood pressure; fasting glucose of >100 mg/dL; triglyceride levels of >150 mg/dL; HDL levels < 40 mg/dL for men and < 50 mg/dL for women. Note that physical *inactivity* and not too much activity (wear and tear) is the fundamental issue. If there is a fracture of the joint surface or severe damage to stabilizing ligaments, posttraumatic arthritis might ensue. But the vast majority of cases of joint disease is not from that. In prehistoric times, for instance, there was definitely a lot of trauma, but not nearly as much joint disease.[14] Another myth I should dispel is the one that has you believing that obesity comes *after* your arthritis or pain and the excess energy storage is the fault of bum joints. In truth, obesity *precedes* arthritis in most cases.[15] Connective tissue diseases of the joints take decades to develop; they don't just happen suddenly.[16] So, the lack of movement is more relevant to our problems than too much movement.

As a people, we collectively sit rather than move. When we cook meals, our ingredients, utensils, and appliances require us to walk fewer than five feet in any direction in our kitchen. When we need galoshes, gadgets, or groceries, we order them online to be delivered to our door. When we want entertainment, we *watch* a sporting event, *watch* children play, or *watch* the stock market rise and fall. If something needs repair, we skip the self-help effort and call in experts. At home, when we wash our wrinkle-free clothes (rather than walk outside to hang them to dry), we toss them into the washer, then the dryer, and then put them away. At work, we sit at a desk, handle paperwork, or phone a friend for a favor.

I'm sure you've heard the ubiquitous refrain from health-care workers: "Sitting is the new smoking." Researchers who analyzed thirteen studies of sitting and lack of activity found that those who sat for more than eight hours a day without physical activity had a risk of dying similar to the risks posed by smoking. The same research shows that sitting increases your risk of premature death from *all causes* just as much as smoking does. In addition to the very real risk of blood clots, sedentary people have higher blood sugar, higher blood pressure, higher bad cholesterol (LDL), and a slower lymphatic system (as it moves waste products out of your system) than people who routinely exercise.[17]

Sitting slows your blood flow, often causing blood to pool in your legs. You may have attended a wedding where a groomsman or bridesmaid passed out while standing in one spot for a long time. (Even the guards at Buckingham Palace are told to stand on their toes frequently to prevent this pooling of blood in their legs.) People with varicose veins and swollen legs or ankles can often blame sitting and poor circulation for the problem.

Why are we so sedentary as a group? For starters, we fear pain. We become focused on what hurts rather than how to make the pain stop with movement. Many physicians still tell patients to avoid activity when they complain of pain. We socialize over Zoom. Everything is delivered. Most of us walk nowhere. I remember seeing a report about a coffee shop that used a lot of time and money to find ways to reduce the number of steps workers took each day in the name of efficiency. This was lauded, and the stock price rose. Meanwhile, the health of the workers suffered further.

Another reason people ignore exercise: they misunderstand its purpose. Exercise isn't about looking good or losing weight. If 5 to 10 percent of body weight is lost with portion control, cartilage loss can be stopped.[18] In my opinion, the *real* purpose of exercise is to make you feel better, increase energy, improve the function of your body, and prevent conditions like dementia and heart disease.

FLEXIBILITY TO KEEP FUNCTIONING

Hip, knee, and back pain typically limit your flexibility and mobility, and in turn increase joint stiffness. Despite any pain you experience, however, a physical therapist can lead you through specific exercises to stop this downward spiral and restore your range of motion and flexibility. In fact, exercise therapy may outperform surgery in some cases. One study of 140 adults with degenerative medial meniscal tears followed those who underwent twelve weeks of physical therapy versus surgery to repair their knee damage. In a two-year follow-up study, the observed differences in the trial group versus the control group was "minute." Plus, the exercise group showed more positive effects than the surgery group in improving thigh muscle strength.[19]

Jim, an older friend of mine in his late seventies, has people frequently ask him how he stays so physically fit and looks twenty years younger than his age. His standard response: "Keep moving to keep moving." And that's fairly the gist of living well longer: consistent exercise and activity.

Of course, many things can wreak havoc with your skeletal system: falling down stairs, breaking your ankle while jumping on a trampoline with a toddler, a skiing accident, and so on. But barring one of these events, exercise slows the cellular aging process that eventually weakens bones, joints, and muscles. The beautiful system that is your human body must move to maintain itself.

A ROLLING STONE GATHERS NO MOSS

Movement is key. "Use it or lose it" is a real thing. When astronauts go into a zero-gravity environment, they return with osteoporosis. Why? Because the body senses no need for calcium to be in the bone as there is no need for compressive strength without gravity. So the body pulls the calcium out. The same thing happens to your cartilage and connective tissues when you are sedentary most of the time. A joint will actually fall apart quicker from lack of use than from overuse.

One of the greatest things about the body is its plasticity. This means that it can change depending upon exposure. If a muscle is exposed to progressive loads, it becomes stronger. If a bone is exposed to load, it too becomes stronger. One of the absolute best ways to add back bone mass when diagnosed with osteopenia or osteoporosis is to start weight-bearing exercise. The connective tissues, muscle, bone, and even skin can adapt to forces imparted by activity. Even the most sedentary individual has a capacity for change. You are not alone if you don't exercise. Fewer than 5 percent of people meet guidelines for activity.[20] But you can get there. Simply starting is all that is needed. As Lao Tzu said, "A journey of a thousand miles starts with the first step."

You don't have to go to extremes either. A low-dose exercise regimen (five exercises for twenty to thirty minutes) is as effective as a high-dose regimen.[21] I am not going to describe specific protocols for exercise; that falls outside the scope of this book. Rather, I am simply emphasizing the need for movement and lifting heavy objects occasionally. Seek guidance from a professional regarding a particular regimen. But, truly, simply walking and doing a few simple lifts is all that is needed.

BRAIN BRAWN

Several studies have shown that exercise improves your brain.[22] Exercise actually generates new neurons to send information between parts of the brain, and also between the brain and the rest of the nervous system.[23] People with lower bone density have a greater risk of developing dementia. This is linked to sarcopenia (loss of muscle), low vitamin D levels, and age.[24] The common denominator among all of these shared risks is a lack of resistance or load placed on the musculoskeletal system.

Exercise increases the size of your hippocampus (your memory depot). Researchers have found that as it increases in size, the hippocampus creates more connections between brain cells, helping you recall memories and store new memories. According to several studies, even after only six months of exercise, people experience significant increases in their brain's gray and white matter.[25]

Exercise seems to release neurotrophins, innate proteins that support brain plasticity. Brain-derived neurotrophic factor (BDNF) is especially important. BDNF actively supports the survival and growth of many types of brain cells.[26] Exercise is integral to its production and release. For your brain to resist cognitive decline, you must move.[27]

HAPPINESS

You've no doubt heard of the "happy molecules" or the "feel-good" molecules: dopamine, serotonin, endorphins, oxytocin, and cannabinoids. Serotonin, for example, is created from the essential amino acid tryptophan. This amino acid enters your body through your foods and is released into serum by exercise like walking, running, swimming, or biking.[28] After about thirty minutes of such exercise, the serotonin level becomes elevated. Less intense exercise increases your serotonin but not as high or as quickly. Serotonin plays a role in metabolic function of the brain.

These molecules and chemicals in your system regulate your moods and emotions, instructing your body to decrease stress, increase your pain tolerance, and promote a sense of well-being in general.[29] Without these molecules, you may feel increased anxiety and depression. Hostility, a negative emotion, is also reduced with exercise. Hostility is associated with more all-cause deaths.[30]

LONGEVITY

Exercise activates your longevity genes. In one particular study that covered adults of all age groups, 8.3 percent of deaths were attributed to inadequate physical activity. For older adults between the ages of forty to sixty-nine, lack of exercise was a significant cause of death (9.9 percent). For those adults aged seventy or older, 7.8 percent of the deaths were attributed to lack of exercise.[31]

Here's what happens at the cellular level: Researchers investigated the telomeres—structures at the end of a chromosome that decrease in length as we age—in the blood cells of thousands of individuals, both those who exercised routinely and those who did not. The people who exercised frequently had longer telomeres, indicating less cellular aging and a longer life span ahead. According to the Centers of Disease Control and Prevention, individuals who exercise at least 150 minutes a week have a healthier life span by almost a decade.

AEROBIC EXERCISE

Aerobic exercise refers to keeping the big muscles of your body in continuous movement for a period of time: running, biking, swimming, fast walking, rowing. This is when the energy source converts from readily available phosphocreatine and glycogen in the muscle to oxidation of fatty acids using oxygen (oxidative phosphorylation). Aerobic exercise is known to help with all-cause mortality and cardiovascular disease, but it also helps with the everyday aches and pains most of us have.[32]

Exercise will make you feel better and have less pain. Studies show an equivalency between exercise and NSAIDs, acupuncture, and corticosteroid injections, with no side effects.[33]

Don't confuse steady-state aerobic exercise with high-intensity interval training (HIIT) workouts. These are great to support brain health and overall fitness, but they are not intended primarily to develop aerobic fitness. HIIT involves training in short intervals of very intense anaerobic exercise, with brief recovery times between sets. HIIT increases the amount of oxygen your body can use (your VO_2 max) while exercising at peak. It helps to regulate insulin sensitivity and can aid the mitochondria to convert the energy stored in macronutrients. HIIT also improves muscle strength[34] and can help with the pain and functional loss of musculoskeletal conditions.[35] HIIT is for those with exercise experience; while it can be a very efficient method to achieve goals, it definitely requires guidance.

To select the best activities and routines, consider your work schedule, family logistics, medical history, and long-term fitness goals. Don't sabotage yourself by deciding that you're going to the gym every afternoon at five thirty when you know from experience you have to pick up kids from school or that your teen often needs to borrow your car for an after-school job. That's setting yourself up for disappointment or conflict. Too many misses lead to failure in forming an exercise habit. Instead, schedule an exercise program that works for everyone involved at least 80 percent of the time. Also, allow a little warm-up and cooldown time after each intense session.

RESISTANCE TRAINING

Resistance exercise means exactly what it sounds like: Your body pushes and pulls against some sort of resistance—lifting and lowering barbells or independent weights, using resistance bands (long, thick rubber bands), pushing against a wall with your body weight, push-ups, and so forth.

We've discussed the use-it-or-lose-it principle. As you age, your bones lose density, and your muscle mass grows weak and soft. Resistance training (RT) will stop this problem. To have better joints, less pain, more function, and better performance, you must avoid sarcopenia.[36]

Life expectancy is around eighty years old. At least 50 percent of us will reach that age with frailty and sarcopenia. Sarcopenia is a hallmark of most NCDs—it presents as weakness and loss of muscle. Muscle becomes infiltrated with fat, chronic inflammation, oxidative stress, is insulin resistant, and enjoys less blood flow. There is, however, a safe and very effective way to

treat this problem: resistance training, which will allow you to reverse sarcopenia.[37] Your fall risk will drop. You will be able to lift your grandchildren
and clean the house without pain. You will also have better cognition as a
side effect.[38]

Building strength does not mean building bulk. I do not want to be bulky,
but I want to be strong. What strength building requires is progressive over-
load, which forms the basis of RT. This means you start with a heavy weight
that you can handle and increase the load over time. The body is plastic, and it
will change to accommodate the new demands. The demands must happen—
and they must happen consistently. So when you decide to build strength, you
need a commitment. What you don't need is a ton of time.

Once you determine the load you can handle with a given exercise, you
can figure your "one rep max." There are many online calculators for this task,
which is the absolute maximum you can lift a single time. To find it, do an
online search for "one rep max calculator."

For strength training, you would do a particular exercise at about 70 to 80
percent of that load for three to five repetitions. Ideally, you would do three to
five different exercises three to five days a week. It is important to rest between
sets, normally for three to five minutes.[39] It is also important to allow recovery
between workout days. The recovery for strength is paramount because this is
when the muscle is made. During the lifting session, signals are sent out by the
cells that more muscle is needed to adapt to the new circumstances. Protein
takes a few days to build, and the connective tissues must adapt and collagen
must be built as well. So, make sure to have recovery days.

Protein intake is important. It should be about 1 g/kg/day, more if you are
doing resistance training.[40] Most of us will lose 1 to 2 percent muscle mass each
year starting at age forty. Through different pathways, resistance training and
protein consumption induce muscle synthesis.[41]

My advice would be to get an appointment with a physical therapist or
personal trainer to get started. Your best bet is an individualized program that
you will enjoy.

Strength is your best weapon against all orthopedic conditions.

STRETCHING

If you have a sedentary life at work and home, then stretching is a must to keep your muscles flexible and pain-free. Stretching, alongside exercise, builds tissue tolerance. As we've said all along, your body and mind are totally integrated. So when you feel stressed, your muscles get tense—in your neck, shoulders, and back. Stretching your muscles purposefully and gently relaxes them, ultimately releasing the stress.

A yoga class works well for stretching. But you can also just stretch wherever you are and whenever you think of it. If you've been hunched over looking at your phone or desk, stand up and bring the shoulder blades together. Whatever your common daily position is, try to counteract it on a daily basis. Stretching can reduce pain from your contracted tissues.[42]

Keep these general guidelines in mind about stretching:

- Stretch with mindfulness and intention. That is, pay attention to the area you're stretching. Move slowly, gracefully, and with purpose.
- Stretch to the point just before you start to feel discomfort, then release the muscle.
- Hold each stretched position as long as you can comfortably do so. Remember that your goal in stretching is to add stress to the muscle and then relax as you release it. All of your connective tissues will adapt to these movements over time.
- Breathe naturally and smoothly through your nose, not your mouth.
- Inhale and exhale deeply to relax and release the stretched muscle.
- Stop stretching if you ever feel dizzy, short of breath, or severe pain.

Chapter Five

OPTIMIZE WITH DIET

Weight loss doesn't begin in the gym with a dumbbell; it starts in your head with a decision.

—Toni Sorenson

Why are 50 percent of all Americans either overweight or obese? Why do 90 percent suffer from metabolic dysfunction? Believe me, there's plenty of blame to go around for this health blunder. For starters, most people think their diets are relatively healthy and have no reason to change. Each day in my clinic I see a complete lack of insight as to how bad for us the American diet is, as provided and promoted by the food industry. You're not alone if you think you're eating well. Many make the same mistake. Most of my patients are not aware that Bunny Bread might be bad for them!

People who have poor diets typically know and admit it. But people who think they're eating healthy are usually wrong.

But don't blame yourself. Instead, consider the goals of the food industry. Like all other businesses, food and beverage companies want to make money so they can meet their overhead. No surprise there. Just beware of what's happening to your body when you fall for the bait and choose to eat a delicious bag of chips. By the way, it is nothing new that the food industry is trying to destroy our bodies in a very slow and methodical fashion. In the 1900s, the Armour Company put formaldehyde in rotted meat in order to feed it to us! Likewise, the term *swill*, which denotes something awful, began when the milk industry fed dairy cows the waste from breweries (swill) in the 1850s. The cows were closely confined, in filthy conditions. Often, these cows stood in their own feces their entire lives as they were bitten by hordes of insects. Sadly, the *New York Times* reported that eight thousand babies died from this milk in one year.[1]

THE FOOD INDUSTRY HAS FOOLED US

Analyses of sugar-industry-sponsored documents as far back as the 1960s and 1970s suggest that their research programs successfully cast doubt about the hazards of sucrose (sugar). They instead blamed fat as the primary culprit in causing coronary disease.[2] Indeed, there was a scientific battle during the time between the major proponent of fat as the villain (Ancel Keys) and sugar as the true villain (John Yudkin). The fat team won and, for a very long time, we have focused on fat alone as the cause of poor health. We know a lot more now, but even so the US population still consumes more than 300 percent of the recommended daily amount of added sugar.[3]

Both the food industry and the federal government seem to admit that they have created the worldwide obesity epidemic. Yet, it's untrendy to discuss this phenomenon, because some people will likely accuse you of fat shaming. Such accusations, of course, are by design. (To be clear, there is nothing healthy for a human about the storage of excess energy in and on the body.) Unfortunately, it seems that few people in powerful positions want Americans or global citizens to take control of their own health and wellness. Rather, the elite and the powerful in corporations and government want to make our food choices *for us* and sell us their healthcare treatments. However, the industry is sensing the groundswell of interest in better foods. Therefore, they will now give us branded "natural" foods! Whew!

In fact, the government created a public-private partnership to reimagine or reformulate the highly processed foodstuffs on grocery store shelves. But reformulating is not the answer we need—processed food labeled "natural" is often still processed. We as citizens must demand healthier food in our stores and restaurants—not just a *different* set of bad ingredients. There's no doubt that ultraprocessed and ready-to-consume foodstuffs are a major cause of most modern health problems. The evidence is overwhelming, but often disregarded. Simply altering a few aspects of packaged food made in a factory does not change it from a synthetic mess to whole food.

We grew up with the food pyramid. This has changed a bit over the years. However, the premise is that we are supposed to eat certain amounts of certain groups of macronutrients. Today's cutting-edge nutrition scientists are working on a far more useful way to think about food. Much of the early and best work has emerged from South America, particularly from Brazil.

For purposes of our discussion here before we get into the specifics, consider a simple classification of foods, as proposed by Dr. Carlos A. Monteiro:[4]

Group 1: Fresh, whole, or minimally processed foods
Group 2: Culinary ingredients; foods obtained directly from group 1
Group 3: Ready-to-consume, processed foods
Group 4: Ultraprocessed foods

The best choices for your diet? In my opinion, this is very simple. Cook your own whole foods at home. (No, that's not frying eggs and sausage for breakfast, grilling sirloin steaks with hot rolls for dinner, or making a milkshake for a bedtime snack.) Also, reheating a prepackaged meal doesn't count. The number of additives and chemicals and processing required to make it shelf-stable renders that meal useless or even harmful to your health. In my opinion, this also includes pre-packaged diet meals.

In my opinion, we shouldn't worry so much about consuming 15 percent fats and 40 percent carbs, for instance. Instead, we should be concerned about whether you ate something whole and real, or did you just eat a fake foodstuff created in a lab and made in a factory with an unhappy labor pool? What I'm telling you goes against most common dietary and nutritional advice. But I live and practice in the real world. Nobody I know has time and energy to count percentages of macronutrients and such. It's much more effective to simply go for real substances that can be easily found and prepare them yourself. You almost can't help but eat a proper ratio of everything that way. Granted, some people need specific diets for specific reasons, such as those suffering from illnesses like cancer or epilepsy. But, in general, if you just follow the traditional Mediterranean way of life, you'll feel a lot better, be more flexible, and enjoy a better life. When you combine this with an approach known as time-restricted eating, which we will discuss more later, you will really be firing on all cylinders.

The first rule of the Mediterranean protocol is to avoid ultraprocessed foods.

WHAT IS ULTRAPROCESSED FOOD?

Ultraprocessed foods—factory-made foodstuffs—usually contain one or more toxic ingredients, or ingredients that can be toxic in certain quantities. Examples of these include sugars, high-fructose corn syrup, trans fats, advanced-glycated-end-products (AGEs), nitrates, pesticides, emulsifiers, coloring, stabilizers, and more. It is important to stress that the traditional processing of food in and of itself is rather harmless. Minimal processing extends the life of a product that's fresh from the source. Whole foods that are dried, salted, frozen, to make them stable and last longer are still okay to consume (e.g., dried chickpeas, dried fruit, pickled vegetables, smoked salmon). It is instead the ultraprocessing methods perfected by mass production engineers that create the harmful final food product. I have a rule you could try at home as well: if a loaf of bread can last for a month without molding, you probably don't want to eat it if you have the choice.

Such ultraprocessed foods are created by deconstructing real food into pieces and parts, and then reconstructing them following specific engineering guidelines. A lab puts together a group of molecules to end up looking and tasting like "food." Factories actually *engineer* these foods like sweet or salty snacks to become addictive. In fact, some manufacturers even advertise their addictive nature with jingles like, "Bet you can't eat just one!"

The NOVA classification defines ultraprocessed this way: "Formulations typically with ≥ 5 ingredients including those also used for food processing itself, such as sugar, oils, fats, antioxidants, stabilizers, emulsifiers, colorants, and preservatives. Ingredients only found in ultraprocessed products include substances not commonly used in culinary ingredients and additives whose purpose is to imitate sensory qualities of group 1 foods or of culinary preparations of these foods, or to disguise undesirable sensory qualities of the final product."[5] Scary, right? In other words, an ultraprocessed food is designed to imitate a real food. But it is not real food. These foodstuffs are one of the main reasons your body does not feel right.

Proteins are hydrolyzed or enzymatically denatured. Starches are broken apart and modified, then enriched with synthetic micronutrients. The same is true of different flours. Food factories use processed and refined oils heavy in omega-6 polyunsaturated fats or even trans-fats. Fats become trans fats during a hydrogenation process that converts a normally liquid oil to a solid oil at room temperature. This process stabilizes a product, increasing its shelf life. Any food that has a partially hydrogenated oil has trans fat by definition. Then the factory combines the fats with sugars and processed syrups designed to tempt your sweet tooth and lower your resistance.

Bleaches, solvents, and salt are used liberally in the engineering of the final food product. Only the cheapest ingredients are used in the mass-produced factory-food/fast-food products. Different chemicals, colors, and textures are added to mimic the tastes, textures, and smells of real food. For example, frozen pizza, pasta dishes, burgers, chips, canned meats, and many canned vegetables. As a result of all this careful engineering, ready-to-eat or ready-to-cook foods often resemble the real thing—but you are basically eating counterfeit food.

I suggest that you avoid packaged food with more than five or six ingredients if possible. Clearly, it's impossible to avoid these all the time, which is why I am such a believer in antioxidants and natural anti-inflammatories, which provide a way to protect yourself from the onslaught of these products. Ultra-processing causes an increase in chronic low-grade inflammation and oxidative stress (free radicals) in the body. When you eat such food, you must have a defense system in place.

Research teams point out that fast foods might meet the criteria for substance dependence (addiction) as defined by the American Psychiatric Association (APA)—"a cluster of cognitive, behavioral, and physiological symptoms indicating continued use of a substance despite significant substance-related problems. There is a pattern of repeated substance ingestion resulting in tolerance, withdrawal symptoms if use is suspended, and an uncontrollable drive to continue use." While these same researchers conclude that the concept of fast-food addiction remains to be proven, the findings of their study support the idea that fast food is potentially addictive and most likely creates dependence in vulnerable groups of people.[6] Fast food is the ultimate form of ultraprocessed foodstuffs. Sadly, this country celebrates fast food and the billionaires who make such products easily available to average citizens. Notably, the APA does not list sugar in their group of substances that cause dependence. If you have a sweet tooth (aka sugar addiction), you know that you have substance dependence. We should all realize this and treat it as such.

According to another research team, these engineered, addictive foods have several things in common. They are (1) high in energy density and low in volume; (2) easy to eat quickly; and (3) highly flavorful.[7] We know now from many functional MRI scan studies and basic science research that the brain changes from the use of added sugar in similar ways to using hard street drugs. Ultraprocessing is the only way to create addictive, dangerous, and shelf-stable foodstuffs that humans crave.

How do UPFs harm us? For starters, there is some evidence available that ultraprocessing of food is associated with elevated levels of glycated hemoglobin (HbA1C) and higher levels of CRP. That association is less meaningful when body mass index (BMI) is factored.[8] By definition, ultraprocessed foods are of poor quality, lack micronutrients, lack fiber, have added sugars and fats along with high energy density. The function of your immune cells is dramatically reduced by the effects of these foodstuffs.

By eating UPFs, you are creating an internal environment that is proinflammatory, pro-oxidant, and proadvanced glycation. None of this works well for your joints, tendons, ligaments, muscle, bone, and connective tissues (or your brain and heart for that matter).

It's noteworthy that your body can process and eliminate such factory foods if you eat them only *occasionally*. But the problem is that almost *all* of our modern Western diet includes ultraprocessed foods. Something like 80 percent of the US diet is highly or ultraprocessed. After all, who invites a coworker or client out to lunch for a quick bite of broccoli? I get it—you won't eliminate all chips, french fries, and so on, from your diet. I probably won't either. The key is to be as healthy as you can on a regular basis. When you do eat a fake food, your body will be far more equipped to detoxify afterward.

Prior to the twentieth century, most food was minimally processed or altogether unprocessed. Meals and dishes were created from whole food and only changed through cooking, which included the addition of spices, salt, or pepper. These meals represented a social gathering, and the entire process of meal creation was celebrated. In some countries today, you'll find this still true, but it's rapidly disappearing as a family tradition.

Now, most people consume ready-to-eat, packaged products and then snack on packaged "treats" throughout the day. The art and beauty of food has disappeared (except maybe in fine-dining restaurants) and has been replaced by meals that degrade our bodies and health.

If you're ever in doubt about whether a food has been ultraprocessed, ask yourself this question: Did it exist two hundred or even one hundred years ago? If not, it's probably processed. (For reference, the Cheeto was invented in 1948. This could be the finest testament to perfectly engineered foodstuffs ever. Who doesn't love Cheetos?)

WHAT'S NONPROCESSED FOOD?

Our nonprocessed food comes from a variety of sources:

Animals: Fresh meat, seafood, milk, and eggs. We generally eat these fresh items soon after slaughter, farming, or tending the source.

But we must be aware, however, that many animal products are heavily processed prior to even reaching the butcher. Beef cattle, for instance, are placed into highly concentrated feed lots toward the end of their lives and then fed vast amounts of corn and soy products. This makes the beef full of fat and omega-6 polyunsaturated fatty acids (PUFAs). Grass-finished (fed grass 100 percent of its life) beef has less omega-6, less fat, and more omega-3 PUFAs. I try to only eat grass-finished beef when I eat red meat. Chicken presents similar problems—think of chickens that are bred for breasts so large they are unable to stand. Farm-raised fish are also often fed a mixture of corn meal and rendered fish, with high concentrations of omega-6 oils, fundamentally changing the nature of the seafood. This farm-raised fish is no longer a healthy product and not a strong source of omega-3 oils. When shopping for fish, it's important to look for wild caught only.

Plants: Leaves, stems, tubers, roots, nuts, seeds, and fresh fruits. If these are frozen, chilled, or vacuum packed, consider them unprocessed or minimally processed. To be classified as minimally processed, a food should not have anything added or removed from it that would significantly change its nature. For example, minimal processing includes cleaning, hulling, peeling, scaling, drying, pasteurizing, malting, fermenting, refrigerating, salting, or vacuum packing the food. To avoid spoiling or molding, minimal processing a fresh food can allow for some preservation or storage—to make it last slightly longer or make it easier to cook and digest. Frozen vegetables are an interesting case in that they are sometimes even better for us than fresh ones. Today, vegetables are picked, blanched, and frozen on the spot. This ensures that all the phytonutrients are locked into the product.[9]

Culinary Ingredients: Because food also meets our social and emotional needs, the culinary ingredients matter. To prepare and cook safe, delicious meals, we use culinary ingredients such as oils, fats, sugar, flour, salt, pepper, garlic, and other spices. Dishes that include these ingredients are still minimally processed and yet long-lasting. Simple processes (milling, pulverizing, crushing, grinding, and pressing) developed hundreds or thousands of years ago help us create culinary staples.

If you need "proof in the pudding" about healthful processing methods, consider this: In societies that still use culinary ingredients and honor these culinary traditions using unprocessed or minimally processed foods, obesity and chronic disease are rare. Remember: processing has been around forever—since humans had fire. Most foods need some sort of processing to make them safe to eat and last longer than a day or two. It is the factory-made-food industry's ultraprocessed products that damage your body and brain.

HAS THE FDA FAILED US?

The process for approvals for food products, food additives, and processing chemicals is similar to that for drugs. Once a drug gets approved by the Food and Drug Administration (FDA), the marketing push begins to promote the drug to get as many products sold as quickly as possible. Time is the enemy. First, patent exclusivity lasts for only a set number of years after the time taken for regulatory requirements—typically ten years—before a generic can be approved. Second, the FDA approves drugs for acute use only for a six-week period. So, drug companies don't really have to prove long-term safety or effectiveness. And according to a recent study published in the *Journal of American Medical Association*, only an astonishing 39 percent of the drugs approved in the FDA's accelerated program have any therapeutic value at all![10] The challenge for these companies is to produce and sell as many products as possible before any potential health hazards or side effects surface, and before the patent expires.

One glaring example of how our regulators missed the ball is high-fructose corn syrup (HFCS). Most health advocates tell you to avoid this sweetener, just as you should avoid any added sugar, yet Americans still eat a ton of the stuff. Our USDA subsidizes the corn farming industry, and this is a cheap and abundant source of added sweetness for our foods. The FDA states that HFCS is generally recognized as safe (GRAS). It isn't even considered to be an additive! Meanwhile, to date, the FDA is still saying that CBD is harmful. In fact, as of January 2023, the FDA has announced they think CBD is so dangerous that they will regulate it as if it were a pharmaceutical. No such concern is given to HFCS.

Only in 2015 did the FDA state that partially hydrogenated vegetable oils were not GRAS. As of 2020, they stated that fully hydrogenated rapeseed oils are safe in some products, and industry has moved to use fully, instead of partially, hydrogenated oils and trans fats (as of 2018). However, I think you know that all the added fats to make processed foods last for months on a shelf are not so good for your body.

Consider the cycle: Such foods create metabolic problems that the pharmaceutical companies then "treat," and insurance companies then "cover" people suffering from chronic diseases caused by poor foods from the food and beverage industries. Since none of that really works, the government then spends massive amounts of money on disability payments and such.

The FDA approved olestra as a fat substitute that transits the digestive system without being absorbed. It is an ingredient in many snacks and chips. However, the side effects of olestra include abdominal cramping and diarrhea. This fat substitute also inhibits absorption of vitamins and other nutrients. The FDA has also approved sodium nitrite, potassium bromate, acesulfame-K, and the hydrogenated vegetable oils discussed earlier—all of which, health experts agree, cause harm to the human body. What is in your grocery store has been blessed as something that won't kill or hurt you quickly, but that doesn't mean it will make your joints feel good.

I could go on with the contradictory and controversial approvals, but you get the point: You can't depend on others to keep you safe by allowing only healthy foods and helpful drugs into the marketplace. They may mean well, but the massive lobbying effort put forth by the food industry and pharmaceutical industry is hard to handle. If a significant portion of the budget of a regulatory industry comes from the industry it regulates, it stands to reason that the industry will hold influence.

Today, government agencies around the world are partnering with the food and pharmaceutical industries to create yet more ultraprocessed food to *replace* the current, harmful ultraprocessed foods. Granted, they claim they are reimagining our choices on the grocery store shelves. But simply replacing *current* processed foods with *different* processed foods carries its own potential risks.

Pharmaceuticals and the medical sciences always seem late to the conversation regarding the root cause and prevention of health problems. Wellness and optimal health get ignored. But without the food industry and compliant, even coddling governmental authorities creating harmful products, most doctors (like myself) would be out of their practices. I understand this and actively try to put myself out of business every day. I tell all my patients that if they do what I say, they won't have to come see people like me anymore!

The entire health-care industry rests on the production of chronic inflammation, advanced glycated end products (AGEs), and oxidative stress within our bodies. Without chronic inflammation and oxidative stress, we'd have few chronic diseases. But we do. So, physicians continue to react and treat the symptoms every day. That's also how a very large portion of the government's budget gets spent each year. Government-run insurance. Medicare. Medicaid. Disability. Research on cures for conditions created by terrible food, stress, pollution, and lack of sleep. Note that no insurance program, including Medicare, will help you pay for supplements, yoga classes, or grass-finished beef.

To date, there's no actual scientific evidence that changing the engineering formula of a given product to make it "healthier" is actually improving the population's health. Yes, a few studies show that a forced reduction of sodium in foods may actually lead to a drop in blood pressure. But those results are probably related to a simultaneous drop in sugar consumption. This marketing trick of simply relabeling foods just allows even deeper penetration of harmful foods into the population. In fact, if you compare the labels of many "healthy" and "natural" protein bars, you will find that they are not that different from a candy bar. Try that one day at the store. It's quite a disappointment.

Don't be duped. You will not get cholera from drinking water, and you should not get salmonella or listeria from foods. However, you will also not get "health" from our current group of foodstuff products available in most of the stores. This is particularly true for those that do most of their shopping in convenience stores—as many of our underprivileged do.

MEDICAL SCHOOLS HAVE FAILED US

With regard to nutrition, the medical industry is particularly inept. Only 13 percent of medical schools teach nutrition. Instead, students learn pharmacology, organic chemistry, and physiology. Rarely do they study psychosocial issues.

Prior to the nineteenth century, the awareness of macronutrients (fats, proteins, carbohydrates) did not fully exist. Once these elements of food were identified and understood, nutrition science focused on them. Later, the medical world also caught on to the fact that micronutrients were important. However, most of the medical treatment of nutrition-based diseases focused on deficiencies and certainly not on optimal health.

For example, for vitamin D deficiency, most of the concern was to prevent rickets—not to improve optimal bone health and optimal immunity. Finally, as a result of the initial work by Ancel Keys in his seminal *Seven Countries Study* (1978), and many who followed, we now realize the importance of micronutrients and macronutrients as potential treatments for our noncommunicable chronic diseases.[11]

The scientific man does not aim at an immediate result. He does not expect that his advanced ideas will be readily taken up. His work is like that of the planter—for the future. His duty is to lay the foundation for those who are to come, and point the way.

—NIKOLA TESLA

PRINCIPLES OF THE MEDITERRANEAN DIET

The Mediterranean diet (that's "diet" with a little *d*) is not actually a diet—a list of approved foods. Instead, think of the Mediterranean diet as a lifetime eating plan, focusing on good, better, and best choices for healthy living. This method of living was named "Mediterranean" by Antonia Trichopoulou and Anna Ferro-Luzzi, and was only later popularized by others.[12]

As you know, there's no single way that all people in the Mediterranean region eat. Rather, populations vary in the amount and type of proteins, oils and fats, alcohol, vegetables, fruits, cereals, breads, nuts, and legumes that they eat. Likewise, the timing of their meals and frequency of exercise vary as well.

Even the studies themselves differ in their scientific methods. Dietary studies are difficult to design and often involve survey data about what people eat, relying on their memory. So, there's controversy around specific foods: Should I or should I not eat this? If so, how often and how much? It's best to avoid discussions about different types of diets, as many diets create tribes of fanatics; it is their way or the highway. I don't want that sort of adversarial attitude to come into your thinking about what you eat!

In general, however, this Mediterranean lifestyle eating plan makes sense and matches my philosophy of life for patients and their families. It's easy to understand and use, can be affordable, and is actually achievable for most people. Although I love the scientific method and research, if we get down in the weeds on nutrition, it's difficult to ever make a firm decision about a specific food that suits all people everywhere no matter their physiology or lifestyle.

The Mediterranean lifestyle eating plan is a group of recommendations rather than a regimen—it's a guidebook for people interested in longevity and happiness. This lifestyle emphasizes social connections and is probably one of the reasons it works so well for health.

The Mediterranean diet itself is based on a research project launched in 1947, when Ancel Keys asked himself this question: Why are so many middle-aged men, seemingly healthy, suffering heart attacks and dropping dead in the United States? He recruited three hundred executive men to take annual examinations and participate in his long-term follow-up on death rates. Later, he incorporated international data from populations that did not have the same rates of heart disease as we did. Eventually, the landmark Seven Countries Study happened. The countries were chosen for contrasting cultures, risk factors, and health outcomes.

As with many such significant studies, the Seven Countries Study proved controversial at first. Much of the early criticism of the study focused on the authors' conclusions that saturated fats were to blame for ill health. There were other cohort studies at the time that didn't find a link between saturated fats and death. Again, this was the time that Dr. Yudkin wrote his seminal piece *Pure, White and Deadly* (1972), which named sugar as the real cause of cardiovascular disease. In the final analysis, the body of work suggests that total fat intake doesn't really matter at all.

However, there are myriad benefits to the Mediterranean lifestyle that matter more, or at least as much, as dietary fat intake (saturated or not). To be clear, the Mediterranean lifestyle is quite high in fat. These other considerations include flavonoid and phenolic content (natural substances in food plants), micronutrient versus macronutrient intake, stress management, and other aspects of a healthy lifestyle. Currently, we're just now beginning to realize how important these other things are to health and wellness.

Shortly after the Seven Countries Study was published, multiple offshoot studies supported the conclusions of the original study. To date as I write this book, more than ten books and 550 peer-reviewed articles cite this work by Dr. Keys.[13] This was one of the first major epidemiological studies of nutrition and really ushered in the notion that "you are what you eat."

There is abundant evidence that the Mediterranean lifestyle can help people to avoid cardiovascular disease, diabetes, and dementia; it can also help people lose weight. This lifestyle diet helps people escape our cultural influences and medicinal methods to become healthier. Much of the success of the Mediterranean lifestyle for managing noncommunicable chronic diseases (NCDs) is linked to its ability to reduce waist circumference, along with its highly anti-inflammatory and antioxidant nature.[14]

Let me add one caveat about all the research: Recall studies form the basis of most dietary literature. These studies require participants to recall *after the fact* what they ate. I don't know about you, but personally, I have difficulty recalling what I ate this morning for breakfast. So I suspect these journal records aren't totally accurate and complete. Generally, however, these studies report that people following the Mediterranean diet eat about 35 to 40 percent of their food as fats, 15 percent from protein, and the remaining 45 to 50 percent from carbohydrates (which includes fruits and vegetables). Don't let your eyes glaze over at these percentages, however. Just note that healthy people consume very limited amounts of saturated fats. Also, carbohydrates are allowed on this diet. It is just that these carbohydrates have a lot of fiber within them. Fiber is one of the keys to ultimate health.

In general, these few core components of the lifestyle eating plan are universal. And even the core principles vary considerably to allow for individual tastes and cultural traditions:

- A high intake of vegetables and fruits: These provide fiber, hydration, and micronutrients
- A high intake of wild-caught seafood, or omega-3 supplementation
- A high intake of cold-pressed extra-virgin olive oil
- Nuts and legumes, minimally processed
- Breads and carbohydrates made from whole grains and unprocessed cereals
- Spices: the antioxidant and phenolic content of spices adds tremendous value with their micronutrients and phytochemicals.
- Healthy omega-3 polyunsaturated fatty acids and fewer omega-6 polyunsaturated fatty acids
- Moderate amounts of dairy items such as milk, eggs, and simply made cheeses—from grass-fed and finished animals
- Limited animal proteins; if the animal is bred naturally, fed natural foods in a cage-free environment, free of toxins and pesticides; grass-finished beef is acceptable
- Limited alcohol

- No refined, processed, added sugars; no fructose unless in a whole fruit
- Few ultraprocessed foods.

The most important part of this lifestyle to remember is to not stress out about it. Just try to eat only foods that you find in nature. Try to cook them at home, with extra-virgin olive oil or avocado oil. Don't add sugar. Try to socialize with friends and family. Take a walk after dinner.

FOODS AND INGREDIENTS

Salt

The latest Dietary Guidelines for Americans recommends that people consume less than 2,300 milligrams (2.3g) of sodium per day. That's one teaspoon. Other studies suggest intake as high as 3,000 to 5,000 milligrams per day.[15] (That's two teaspoons.) Iodized salt (iodine added to salt) ensures you have an adequate supply of iodine. Some researchers insist that too much sodium increases the risk for high blood pressure, heart disease, and stroke. On the other hand, cardiovascular research scientist James DiNicolantonio has concluded that insulin resistance is a much more important predictor of high blood pressure than salt. Once insulin resistance has been reversed, then salt has little, if any, effect on blood pressure.[16] Many health advocates and longevity experts have no problem with six to nine grams of salt each day, assuming you have healthy kidneys. The human kidney is a remarkable machine and will balance your sodium levels all day every day.

Of course, nobody goes to the utensils drawer and pours themselves one to six teaspoons of salt. So how do you get all that salt in your system? According to current research, you have very limited control over your sodium intake. Studies suggest that 71 percent of the sodium we eat comes from food prepared outside your home. Only 14 percent of our sodium intake comes from our actual food.[17]

Chocolate

Cocoa is real chocolate. For your chocolate to be healthy, avoid milk fat or solids, and trans fat. As the name implies, dark chocolate is dark. Many American candies are made with milk chocolate, which is lighter in color. According to European guidelines, dark chocolate must contain at least 43 percent cocoa to be called dark chocolate. For the best health benefits, look for at least 70 percent cocoa chocolate.[18]

There is some controversy in the chocolate world, however. There have been issues with levels of cadmium and lead in chocolates due to polluted soils tainting the beans.[19] Both of these heavy metals can lead to health issues if you consume them regularly and/or in large amounts. If you consider chocolate an occasional treat, and not a health food, you can lower your risk of exposure and still enjoy some chocolate in your life.

Olive Oil

Extra-virgin olive oil is a real juice (from olives), minimally processed. As the primary dietary fat, olive oil plays a huge role in how the Mediterranean eating plan achieves such positive results. The phytochemicals within olive oil, not found in other oils, also give significant benefits. Olive oil also contains large amounts of monounsaturated and polyunsaturated fats that decrease oxidative stress and inflammation. It also has a high content of oleic acid, which prevents heart disease, reduces cholesterol, and lowers blood pressure. Additionally, olive oil helps with DNA repair and is also associated with less age-related cognitive decline. Olive oil supplementation alone is associated with less pain from arthritis and other musculoskeletal conditions.

Think of olive oil as the foundation of the entire plan. It's medicinal by itself. Measured against the vegan, vegetarian, Asian, or national cholesterol-education diets, the Mediterranean eating plan has a higher fat content than other diets. Olive oil synergizes with the omega-3 PUFAs from either seafood or supplementation. Either alone is not as effective for your health as they are together.

Yogurt

Yogurt has healthy bacteria that fight fungus-related infections, and acts as a probiotic. But you want to avoid the kind of yogurt that has sweeteners and fruit-like additives. Back in the '80s when the American Hospital Association (AHA), American Diabetes Association (ADA), and the US Department of Health and Human Services (HHS) were promoting low-fat diets for health, yogurt sales boomed! But that yogurt was filled with sugar and flavoring to make up for the fat that had been extracted during processing. This made it an added-sugar nightmare foodstuff that only added to the obesity problem. Greek yogurt is a good choice, as it is a minimally processed yogurt, ideally made from whole fat milk. Remember: milk fats are not as bad as you have been led to believe. If you don't like Greek yogurt, you can always supplement to rid yourself of pesky GI infections—or eat garlic to do the job!

Coffee

The benefits of coffee on the brain: a positive impact on neurotransmitters. Studies say that drinking twenty-four ounces (three cups) of coffee a day decreases your risk of Parkinson's by 40 percent and your risk of Alzheimer's by 20 percent. On the other hand, for some people, caffeine causes migraines, breast lumps, stomach upset, nervousness, and irregular heartbeats. With coffee, you'll need to decide whether its benefits or dangers concern you the most. Decaffeinated coffee may be your answer. Coffee should be organic and fair trade if possible. That is not always possible, so at least find a source that won't mix in sawdust, twigs, corn, soy, and other additives for volume.[20]

Alcohol

The Bill and Melinda Gates Foundation funded the largest study done to date on alcohol use. After studying results in 195 countries, here's that summary: "Alcohol use is a leading risk factor for a global disease burden and causes substantial health loss. We found that the risk of all-cause mortality, and of cancers specifically, rises with increasing levels of consumption, and the level of consumption that minimizes health loss is zero."[21]

Others believe that moderate alcohol can assist with lowering blood pressure, reducing dementia, and all-cause mortality. Moderate alcohol use causes hormesis and induces the same stress-response repair systems in the cells that fasting and exercise might. This is all very controversial, of course. What is not controversial is that the decades of research on populations that follow a traditional Mediterranean lifestyle demonstrate amazing health benefits and longer life. This lifestyle happens to include moderate alcohol intake.

In sum, some researchers argue that alcohol keeps your arteries young. But other researchers insist that alcohol has a direct toxic effect on your immune system and your brain cells. So you have to weigh the facts and decide what risks you want to take.

Fats

You need both carbohydrates and fats in your diet. Both the quality and quantity of fats affect good health. Healthy fats actually help to stabilize your blood sugar. Just make sure you're eating good fats (olive oil, avocados, nuts, fatty fish, full-fat dairy products such as nonsweetened Greek yogurt).

People where I live in the deep South typically have terrible diets. My theory about why most haven't died by age fifty? Spice! Everything is heavily spiced—particularly with onions, chives, leeks, scallions, garlic, green pepper, bay leaves, black pepper, oregano, rosemary, turmeric, saffron, sage, paprika, parsley, cayenne, and cooked with olive oil. Spices change how your body reacts to fats. People here in the South also have very deep community and family connections, and this too is part of a traditional Mediterranean lifestyle and contributes to lower cortisol levels overall.

Sugars

Eating sugar is just like opening a vein and pouring in poison. Avoid simple sugars like corn syrup, maltodextrin, barley malt, molasses, corn sweetener, brown sugar (and any ingredient ending in -ose). Also skip most white, processed foods. Pay attention to beverages, which is where recent research suggests that we obtain all that sugar. Fully 43 percent of the sugar in our diets comes from beverages. The other 57 percent comes from all other foods combined.[22]

When your blood is high in sugar, that affects the cells lining your blood vessels and arteries, which then leads to inflammation and plaque buildup. Excess sugar also causes more AGEs to form in your tendons and joints. I would refer you to Robert Lustig's book *Sugar Has 56 Names: A Shopper's Guide* for a guide on translating labels.

Artificial Sweeteners

Noncaloric artificial sweeteners were considered safe in the past simply because of their low- or zero-calorie content. But supporting scientific data remains sparse and controversial. The negatives: The sweeteners drive glucose intolerance because of their alterations to the intestinal microbiota.[23] There is a growing body of evidence that points to the alteration of the gut biome in general with these substances. Sucralose has been studied extensively and is considered to be safe. However, there is no consensus as to whether we should avoid these or not. I would submit that added sugar and fructose are probably worse.

Pasta

Low-carb diets have long steered us away from pasta, insisting it was bad for health, but scientific evidence does not support this perception. Most dry pasta is enriched with iron, riboflavin, thiamine, and folic acid. It's also an excellent source of vitamin B. Other things going in its favor: it's inexpensive, convenient, versatile, and filling. Overall, it's wholly compatible with the Mediterranean diet.[24] Pasta usually has a terrible ratio of carbohydrates to dietary fiber, so make sure to eat it with plenty of fiber (vegetables), fats, and proteins to limit the glucose spike and insulin spike that might follow.

I encourage you to follow the big picture principles of healthy eating for a lifetime: Choose fresh, whole foods or minimally manipulated whole foods, sourced locally, and cook them yourself at home. Cooking methods matter a great deal. How you cook meat can make a huge difference in the related cancer risks. Frying, broiling, grilling, and broiling meats at very high temperatures forms chemicals that lead to a cancer risk and more AGEs. On the other hand, stewing, steaming, or braising meats produce fewer of these dangerous chemicals.

HOW WILL THIS HELP MY ARTHRITIS?

There is a large and growing body of knowledge as to the benefits of diet to treat arthritis and other musculoskeletal problems. Pain, generally, is also manageable with better diets.

Let's discuss the current science and thinking regarding diet, pain, and arthritis here.

Soy is now known to produce pain relief. It is antioxidant and anti-inflammatory. It is a great source of protein, equivalent to animal protein, with all the essential amino acids. I often tell my older patients who are frail and have sarcopenia to start eating edamame every day.[25]

Anthocyanins from berries are well known to be associated with a reduced risk of cardiovascular disease, cancer, and other NCDs. These are a phytochemical that has antioxidant and anti-inflammatory properties. For example, tart cherry extract is a very potent antioxidant and has a proven capacity to reduce pain. Cyanidin (from tart cherries) works better than aspirin for inflammation. Also, different compounds in this fruit also reduce the activity of the COX-1 and COX-2 enzymes, much like ibuprofen or naproxen. However, eating tart cherries or supplementing with the extracts does not have the same side effect profile as the chemical NSAIDs.

Arthritis is a whole-joint disease that involves inflammation. During the inflammatory process, the tissues produce immune mediators like cytokines that damage cartilage tissues and cause pain. The Mediterranean lifestyle has very strong anti-inflammatory properties and will reduce the levels of components of the painful arachidonic acid cascade (inflammation) and the expression of certain genes that induce more inflammation. It will also modulate the activity of immune cells. All of this contributes to better outcomes and reduced symptoms of arthritis, tendinitis, and other musculoskeletal diseases.

We know now that higher levels of systemic, low-grade inflammation that cause rapid atherosclerosis also cause arthritic conditions. There is a 50 percent higher risk of cardiovascular disease in those with rheumatoid arthritis than in others. There is also a higher risk with other inflammatory conditions, like psoriasis and gout.[26] In one of the offshoots of the Seven Countries Study, the ATTICA Study, researchers showed that adhering to the Mediterranean lifestyle led to lower uric acid levels and fewer cases of hyperuricemia.[27] We know today that uric acid is not simply a marker for gout, but it might also be causal for a host of NCDs.

When you cook whole foods at home, you will often add spices and other culinary ingredients. As noted earlier, spices themselves are a part of the health benefits of the Mediterranean way and are basically functional foods that act in a medicinal fashion. We will discuss spices in more detail later.

The Mediterranean diet also gives you a better omega-3-to-omega-6 ratio in your cell membranes as an important way to modulate the damage induced by inflammation. This balance is very important regarding the development of chronic diseases like arthritis.

Extra-virgin olive oil (EVOO) contains monounsaturated fatty acids that are anti-inflammatory. In addition, first cold-pressed oils are replete with antioxidants. Oleic acid, oleuropein, and hydroxytyrosol are components of the oil and modify the expression of genes responsible for inflammation such as NF-kB. EVOO has been proven to restore the lubricin levels in animal cartilage even after resecting the ACL.[28] Olive oil applied topically or orally has also shown significant benefits for osteoarthritis.[29] Those who eat fewer fruits and vegetables have a higher risk of developing inflammatory arthritis.[30] A healthy Mediterranean diet will also improve your DNA-methylation parameters, or your epigenetic profile. By improving your epigenetics, you will have less osteoarthritis (along with other NCDs).

With adherence to this dietary pattern, there is also a lower risk of symptomatic osteoarthritis.[31] Data from the Osteoarthritis Initiative also demonstrated a lower prevalence of knee osteoarthritis with adherence to the diet. These outcomes were attributed to the anti-inflammatory aspects of the diet, since inflammation directly contributes to the destruction of cartilage. Likewise, there is less oxidative stress damage to the cartilage. The extracellular matrix of cartilage and connective tissues also functions better with this diet than with a normal diet. In my opinion, this is likely due to fewer AGEs.

When comparing a low-fat diet to the Mediterranean diet, the latter is more effective at decreasing pain. Weight loss was the same between the groups, but people feel better and experience less pain on a Mediterranean diet. This suggests that the pain of knee osteoarthritis relates not to weight, but rather to inflammation.[32] This dietary pattern is as good as NSAIDs for pain reduction.[33]

There is an inverse relationship between how many fruits and vegetables one eats and how many symptoms of osteoarthritis one has. This is true even for the radiographic appearance of osteoarthritis. Eating nine servings per day (in line with the Mediterranean diet) leads to a 46 percent reduction in severe knee pain. Eating between five and nine servings daily led to a 33 percent reduction in severe knee pain. Just two servings of fruit per day led to fewer complaints of pain overall.[34] Think about this: I can't think of a single surgery or drug with such a great track record and no side effects. In a study that found no benefit from vegetables, the authors classified french fries as a vegetable.[35]

The data is clear that you will feel better if you eat a high-quality, Mediterranean style diet.

Yes, fresh whole foods cooked at home help keep you healthy. It's that simple to rid yourself of chronic inflammation that produces aches and pains and to prevent serious diseases and conditions.

TAMING THE OBESITY BEAST?

Over the last few decades, the body of knowledge that pertains to circadian medicine has grown rapidly. One of the original studies that looked at circadian-based feeding times proved the importance of this concept. Scientists had two groups of mice, and both were fed a diet mimicking the standard American diet, fed to lab mice when scientists intended to give them a metabolic disorder, such as diabetes. One group could eat their food whenever they felt like it. The other group was limited to feeding during a short period of the active part of their day. The scientists found that even with a terrible diet, if the mice ate only for a part of the day—and if it was during their normal active time of day—they did not become fat or sick![36] Since then, further proof of the power of what we call time-restricted eating, or TRE, has been found.

The important thing to understand is that if you *are* overweight or obese, you can change that. And as you do so, you can reverse many orthopedic conditions related to excess weight. You must get healthy if you hope to maintain a normal body weight.

Arthritis is a common comorbidity in obese patients. Obesity contributes to the development and progression of arthritis—to the structural and mechanical problems, as well as to changes in inflammation caused by metabolic syndrome.[37] More than a million hip and knee replacement surgeries are

done each year in the United States, and many are for obese patients.[38] Among the elderly, arthritis of the knee is one of the five leading causes of disability.[39] Approximately 26 percent of the total adult population is projected to have arthritis by 2040.[40]

In addition to the link between obesity and arthritis, the risk of type 2 diabetes increases proportionately to an increasing body mass index.[41] Obesity is also a comorbidity with all the leading causes of death: heart disease, stroke, type 2 diabetes, chronic kidney disease, dementia, Alzheimer's disease, and thirteen types of cancer (colorectal, uterine, kidney, breast cancer in postmenopausal women, adenocarcinoma of the esophagus, liver, gallbladder, pancreas, thyroid, ovary, gastric cardia [a part of the stomach], myeloma [a blood cancer], and meningioma [a type of brain cancer]).[42]

In addition to arthritis, other musculoskeletal disorders linked to obesity include lower back pain and inflammation of the hips, knees, shoulders, and neck. Remember: all these problems occur because of damage to the mitochondria, the cell membranes, DNA, and proteins. This damage is from chronic low-grade inflammation and also from free radicals. This pro-oxidant situation happens when there is excessive energy available from unnatural substances; this is what we must avoid.

It's hard to exaggerate how damaging having constant, excess energy is to your health and lifespan. Excess energy availability prevents the body from cleaning itself up or conducting repair. Brain detoxification, for instance, depends on sleep, but perhaps you are unaware of all the other things the body repairs during sleep. Cartilage, nerves, ligaments, muscles, bones, and many other tissues are also detoxified and repaired during sleep. For this process to really be effective, a fasted state is also necessary. You must not only sleep—but sleep *fasted*. This is why restricting when you eat can really help with your overall medical condition.

Are overweight and obese patients really getting the help they need? Plainly and simply, no! According to researchers, patients who report knee pain get treated for their arthritis—but not the underlying cause. But patients with knee arthritis who lose weight show dramatic improvement in knee pain and other symptoms.[43]

So to be successful in solving both problems—weight and related conditions like arthritis, knee pain, hip pain, and such—pay attention to just two things about your eating habits:

1. Consider *when* you eat—what time of day. Time-restricted eating (TRE) is a fundamental part of this protocol. Your daily eating/fasting cycle influences your metabolism and contributes to obesity and other conditions such as insulin resistance and type 2 diabetes.[44]

2. Choose quality foods like those of the Mediterranean lifestyle and avoid ultraprocessed foods (UPFs).

Simply following these two guidelines can dramatically affect your success in both losing weight and avoiding diseases and conditions that you may develop because of obesity.[45]

MITOCHONDRIA AND FASTING

One of the hallmarks of aging is altered mitochondrial metabolism. The mitochondria produce less and less energy, while, as noted earlier, more and more free radicals cause oxidative stress. If there is a constant supply of too much sugar, fructose, and protein, the mitochondria become overwhelmed and simply stop working properly.

The main purpose of the mitochondria is to produce energy for your cells from what you eat. How well your cells work and survive depends totally on how well your mitochondria work. The importance of their proper functioning can't be overstated. Preserving and generating new mitochondria leads to better health and slows aging. Like any machine, constant maintenance is required, and so you must take care of and maintain your mitochondria. This requires mitophagy—the removal of damaged mitochondria—and mitochondrial biosynthesis—the creation of new mitochondria. These processes cannot occur if there is constant excessive energy and a poor circadian rhythm.

Earlier, we saw how our metabolism functions. Aging reduces the ability of the mitochondria to work properly, and free radicals, a normal byproduct of

energy, also impair the mitochondria. These very damaging molecules must also be managed carefully. As we age, the number of these free radicals exceeds the cells' ability to manage them, and this is when oxidative stress and cell damage occur. This is probably one of the reasons many of my patients tell me that they have pain simply because they are "getting older." They are right, but not for the reason they think. Rather, that age group has simply accumulated enough advanced glycation end products and induced enough oxidative stress and inflammation from poor diet and lifestyle to manifest things like tendinitis, arthritis, sarcopenia, dementia, atherosclerosis, and other serious health problems.

The ability of mitochondria to work properly is further compromised by limiting the amount of maintenance these organelles receive and also providing excessive crude fuel. This, unfortunately, is what our current lifestyle does. We don't sleep well, leading to a poor circadian rhythm, and we eat way too much excess sugar and processed foods. One way to manage this, of course, is to "diet" or restrict calories, but this can lead to micronutrient deficiencies—and it's not fun!

While it can be challenging, calorie restriction causes what's known as "healthy aging," meaning that the cell metabolism improves by that restriction instead of being overwhelmed with too much energy. As you limit calories, healthy new cells are created in response to that stress. This process is a normal survival mechanism for humans. By restricting calories using time (say, fasting for 8–14 hours), you can limit the damage to cell metabolism and reduce cellular aging. Longer fasting periods prove even more effective at slowing the aging process. With calorie restriction, you induce what is called the stress-response system. Sensing a lack of energy, the human cell will batten down the hatches and get to work to improve all cellular functions and efficiencies. This is when autophagy and mitophagy happen. This is when cell membranes and DNA are repaired. This is when misfolded proteins are broken down, recycled, and put to good use. Our bodies developed this ability due to evolution. We have always been faced with starvation, and to survive as a species, our systems had to find a way to handle a lack of nutrients and to self-repair.

With all this in mind, one way by which we could manage everyday aches and pains is to allow a daily fasting period for repair and maintenance.

Intermittent fasting, discussed later in this chapter, provides one way to do this. Time-restricted eating—TRE—is also an excellent approach. By simply limiting your feeding window to eight to twelve hours a day, you can provide a minifast each and every day to help your stress-response system get to work. If you match that window to when the sun goes up and down, you can introduce a good circadian rhythm, leading to better health and wellness. A regular routine for bedtime and awakening, combined with time-restricted eating, is the foundation of my protocol for you. As you adapt to this lifestyle—a change which is not hard to accomplish—you'll naturally experience less pain, be more motivated, and perform better in all aspects of your life. Now, let's take a closer look at TRE.

HOW TIME-RESTRICTED EATING WORKS FOR YOU

Fasting goes back thousands of years as a religious practice for a range of beliefs including Judaism, Christianity, and Islam. Fasting has served numerous purposes: A form of protest (hunger strikes and other protests against injustices). A time of self-denial and reflection to contemplate ethical issues or decisions. And for medical reasons. Hippocrates recommended fasting from both food and drink for patients who had certain symptoms, as did other physicians of his time who considered a loss of appetite during a disease as a natural part of the recovery process.

Fasting to reduce weight and improve health has recently become a popular trend again—and what many physicians have embraced as a boon to wellness and long life.

Time-restricted eating (TRE) is a form of daily fasting, wherein a person eats during a limited, compressed time frame. People who practice TRE eat only during certain hours of the day, and fast during the remainder of the twenty-four-hour cycle. Today, the average American eats for most of the day. Grazing and midnight snacks are common. A large shot of fructose immediately upon awakening is common. We eat therefore for about fifteen or sixteen hours each day. The only time we aren't eating or drinking something is literally when we are asleep.

TRE prevents this. For example, you may eat one or more meals or snacks, but all your food intake happens in six hours—say, from noon until 6:00 p.m. Or you may eat during an eight-hour window—say, from 11:00 a.m. to 7:00 p.m. or from 8:00 a.m. to 4:00 p.m. During this eating period, you can eat meals and snacks. There's no restriction on what you eat or when you eat in this specific window. Of course, you'll realize far more benefit if you combine TRE with quality foods like those recommended in the Mediterranean-lifestyle eating plan.

TRE is based on the circadian rhythm. Our biological or body clock is naturally timed to relate to the circadian rhythm in nature. In fact, we have multiple clocks in all the cells throughout our body. Every cell functions on specific schedules due to these genetic timing mechanisms. These clocks control or regulate metabolic systems that support our bodily functions. Our eating-fasting cycle and our sleep-waking cycle entrain these circadian clocks. It's important to note that not only does the sun turn on your master clock in the brain and then the peripheral clock genes, but when you eat also triggers a gut-based clock. This is why matching your eating cycle to your light exposure matters so much. If the gut-derived clock is different from the sunlight-derived clock, then disarray results.

These clock genes orchestrate how the body metabolizes carbohydrates, proteins, and cholesterol. Clock genes function throughout tissues and regulate almost all functions in your body. A small region of the brain (the suprachiasmatic nucleus, or SCN) located within the hypothalamus acts as the master clock and coordinates the rhythms of the other smaller clocks throughout the body found in the muscles, glands, skin, bones, connective tissue, and the brain. The gut and the feeding-managed clock will affect the liver, pancreas, and other gastrointestinal organs as they alternate between eating and fasting. This clock system works throughout our lifetime, but it can change with age or disease. Coordination is paramount to good health.

Eating sends a primary signal to all the body's clocks to start metabolism. But the nutrients we take in can disrupt the smooth rhythm of these clocks.

That is, eating at irregular times from one day to the next can desynchro-nize the circadian rhythms between the master clock and the other cell clocks. That's why you want to adopt TRE as a lifestyle. It is crucial to introduce a routine, and this will not only reduce your stress but also make this healthy life easier and better. Things get out of sync if you change your eating window from day to day or week to week. The repair, detox, and stress-response func-tionalities depend upon a solid routine.

The benefits of TRE are huge: weight loss, reduction in fat mass, improved heart function, improved insulin circulation, lower blood pressure, better joints, bones, and muscle, and more endurance for activity. All those good things happen even without changing what we eat or how much we eat. More importantly for you and me, pain is reduced, and arthritic conditions are also improved.

And once someone gets into the rhythm of the eating schedule, their appe-tite decreases. In addition to multiple human studies on reduction of symptoms, animal studies suggest that other diseases can be countered by time-restricted eating: autoimmune disorders such as multiple sclerosis or lupus, diabetes, and some cancers.[46]

Multiple studies have proven TRE has major benefits, in addition to weight loss. Adopting one of these eating-fasting patterns even for a brief four-week period results in significant reductions in mean body fat percentage, visceral fat, body fat mass, trunk fat, and stress levels. Participants in these studies reported a significant drop in appetite over time and felt no changes in their quality of their sleep or their quality of life overall.[47] With TRE, you only worry about the time twice a day. You do not spend all day thinking about food and you do not burden your brain with dieting.

INTERMITTENT FASTING HELPS TOO

Intermittent fasting (IF) involves restricting calories for a set period. The fast involves going without any food for a longer time than just a time-restricted window within a single twenty-four-hour day. IF may take several forms. For example, a person might fast for a twenty-four-hour, a forty-eight-hour, or a seventy-two-hour period. Some people routinely practice IF by going without food for one day each week and then eating regular meals the other six days. The most supported practice for health benefits appears to be the one proposed by Valter Longo—a two-five schedule: for two days a week a fast occurs, and food is consumed on the other five.[48]

Other people practice IF by alternating days. For example, they eat normally on Monday, fast on Tuesday, eat on Wednesday, fast on Thursday, and then continue this pattern. That, of course, means that the eating and fasting days change from week to week. As you imagine, this daily alternating pattern can become complicated as you plan your social life: Is this the week I'll be eating or fasting on Friday night?

How does fasting for a long period (three to seven days) actually improve your health? Though it's variable, many believe our energy reserves become depleted after two or three days of fasting. Humans are able to store about 1,600–2,800 calories in the form of glycogen. At that point, your body shifts metabolically from burning sugar to a ketogenic state. Some people can achieve ketosis after just a twelve-hour fast. During nutritional ketosis (NK), your body burns fatty acids and ketones for fuel. There's not a lot of insulin around in the absence of glucose and most will enter a catabolic state. Then, when you eat normally again, your cells rebuild. According to Dr. Dan L. Longo, with the National Cancer Institute, this starvation-feeding cycle triggers a regeneration and self-healing process that reduces your biological age.[49] Nice, right?

The same logic applies here with TRE: You set up a regular system of when you eat and when you fast during a twenty-four-hour period. Then your circadian rhythm adjusts and coordinates the clock cells throughout your body. It's possible to achieve the same health benefits with a very routine protocol for time-restricted eating as it is with intermittent fasting.

As you consider these two methods of dietary manipulation—time-restricted eating and intermittent fasting—don't discount them as new, untested ideas. As you probably know, methods of calorie-restriction and fasting have been studied for at least a century. Back in 1946, Anton Carlson and Frederick Hoelzel at the University of Chicago tested food restriction with rats.

Those rats that got food only every third day lived 15–20 percent longer than the rats eating on a regular daily schedule.[50] This is the work that began our understanding of fasting as it relates to longevity and also to health overall.

Between 2000 and 2020, more than eleven thousand studies on intermittent fasting have been carried out. It is becoming abundantly clear that not only following a circadian rhythm with food intake but also giving the body a fasting period are mandatory for a healthy body and brain.

A side note here while we're talking about fasting: As you adopt TRE, keep hydrated. Fasting doesn't mean you go without water. If you're a woman, your body is about 50 percent water. If you're an adult man, you're lugging around 60 percent water. To prevent dehydration, you need to keep replenishing the water. Even mild dehydration can affect your concentration, memory, and endurance. Keep in mind that each gram of carbohydrate is stored with three grams of water. The initial weight loss of a ketogenic diet is primarily water weight. Replacing water is vital.

How much water do you need? To keep it simple, divide your weight by two. That number represents the number of ounces you need every day. So, if you weigh 160 pounds, you need to drink eighty ounces of water every day. Yes, you do! Here's a simple trick to help: Fill a pitcher every morning with the required ounces. Then pour glassfuls from that pitcher all day until the water's gone.

The primary difficulty in implementing these eating and fasting periods across an entire population comes down to money and convenience. Sound familiar? Consider all the industries that have established practices and financial incentives to maintain the status quo of eating three meals along with snacks every day. The public school system. Agriculture, food processing, food retail, and restaurant industries. Even the healthcare industry itself. Why would these industries want you to eat less? You guessed it: money and resistance to change on any large scale. The status quo bias rules again. In addition, there's no way to patent and sell the idea of TRE or indeed the idea of eating less. I don't think you'll ever hear a resounding call for this. That being said, I think you will see how important time-restricted eating can be for making you feel better and for reducing musculoskeletal problems along with most chronic health conditions.

In my opinion, a daily routine is half the battle, and a crucial part of this protocol. If you can just establish a solid bedtime-and-wake-time cycle and then match that to your feeding window, a lot of your problems will be solved. Granted, changing your daily habits to follow a TRE pattern will be going against the grain, no doubt. Many of my friends and family still roll their eyes and shake their heads at me. But then they also no longer make a big deal about my schedule.

Once you have created a solid TRE window and are used to it, then begin to change the types of foods you eat. The combination of a routine fasting period every day with a great diet pattern during feeding is integral to the success of this protocol.

THE MEDITERRANEAN DIET DELIVERS ENERGY AND PREVENTS DISEASE

When diet is wrong, medicine is of no use.
When diet is correct, medicine is of no need.
—AYURVEDIC PROVERB

With what I am teaching you here—about how to naturally manage pain and handle your orthopedic conditions—you will also find that you will benefit from significant improvements to your overall health. Less chance of dementia, a longer life, and lower incidence of heart disease. You'll be able to play with your grandkids, perform at a higher level at work, be more active—whatever you wish!

Your diet is the single most significant risk factor for premature death and long-term disability.[51] However, as a practicing surgeon I understand that encouraging you to make major changes in your life today to (perhaps) add a few years before your potential demise in twenty to thirty years is a somewhat nebulous, if not meaningless, concept. That said, my goal for my patients has always been to make their lives better. I want them to feel better *now*.

If that fact stuns you, good. Keep that in mind as you read further and contemplate your aching back, rickety knee, bum shoulder, arthritic fingers, diabetes, or memory loss. Yes, diet affects all of these conditions and more, and we'll delve into these interactions as we move along. The body of research regarding positive effects of diet and exercise to eliminate aches, pains, and arthritis progression is large and growing. The outcomes from simply switching to a healthy diet and doing moderate exercise a few times a week have proven to offer as good or better outcomes than from any other treatment. The best thing is that this treatment protocol is entirely in your control—you don't need to rely on physicians.

When the word *diet* surfaces in a conversation, strong negative emotions can often arise. So many people have tried diet after diet, but with no success. And some have been highly successful on specific diets, losing sixty, eighty, or one hundred or more pounds—only to regain the weight in a couple of years. So, it's understandable why *diet* can be a dirty word—a real turnoff. The technical definition is "a special course of food to which one restricts oneself, either to lose weight or for medical reasons." Ugh! That is not my style. I believe in everything in moderation; even moderation itself. You don't want to "restrict" yourself. You just want to live a better life and feel better. I promise you that it is possible.

Also, let's talk about why we even need to diet at all. America has invented and ushered in the global obesity pandemic. Precisely why this is the case is the subject of ongoing debate. Some believe it is chemicals in the food. Others believe it is the ultraprocessing of food or just sugar. Others still believe it is a lack of exercise. I could go on and on; but it seems that there is no simple answer. People used to drink raw milk, eat butter, and eat a lot of red meat and did not become obese. People have always eaten carbs and made bread and such and were never obese. That said, it does seem suspicious that the timing of the obesity era mirrors the timing of the food-industry growth and processed foods with excessive added sugars. Just keep that it mind. Maybe that is all you must avoid.

In my opinion, weight loss should not be the primary motivation for a healthy diet. Sure, you will lose weight by changing to better food choices. But that's not the primary goal for recommending the Mediterranean lifestyle diet. If you focus on a narrow target like a certain percentage of weight loss, that goal begins to change the psychology of what you are trying to accomplish. You really want to be healthy from the inside out. You want to do more, be stronger, have less pain, and feel less stiff. Your weight will comply eventually.

The Mediterranean diet is beneficial for brain health, cardiovascular health, diabetes and cancer prevention, and so many other healthy outcomes, including orthopedics. To my knowledge, there is no FDA-approved pharmaceutical that can do all of this for you. Not that enterprising entrepreneurs aren't trying to get a corner on the market of lifetime health and longevity. However, history and tradition have already provided the ultimate protocol for you to follow and achieve all your health goals.

At its core, a lifestyle of healthy food choices leads to less chronic inflammation, lower oxidative stress, and fewer advanced glycation end products. Granted, those technical terms for what may be happening in your body mean nothing to you now.

Chapter Six

SLEEP MATTERS MIGHTILY

You're probably chronically sleep deprived. According to the National Sleep Foundation, if you're over the age of eighteen, you need seven to nine hours of sleep each night—not four, not five, not six. In the past, sleep researchers occasionally and erroneously reported that "some people" need less sleep—but this is not true. In reality, fewer than a fraction of 1 percent of the population has a particular gene (a subvariant of a gene called BHLHE41, also known as DEC2) that actually provides resilience despite little sleep.[1] But your chances of getting hit by lightning are greater than having that gene in your DNA.

Many of you work two jobs while raising children, do daily chores, and volunteer or attend after-work networking events. With hope, we're all trying to fit some exercise into the day as well. Sadly, without enough sleep, our brains give up and force us to fall asleep. Physicians specializing in sleep disorders call this tendency microsleeps. During these five- or six-second microsleeps, the eyelids partially or fully close. If your brain is chronically sleep deprived, then how can you work on a health mindset or think about meal prep?

Researchers studying how sleep deprivation affects workers discovered that these microsleeps result in catastrophic impairment—a mistake rate 400 percent higher than the eight-hour-sleep control group.[2] After just ten days of getting only seven hours of sleep, the brain becomes as dysfunctional as if it had gone without sleep for a full twenty-four hours.[3] And the worst thing researchers have evidence to support: The sleep-deprived group severely underestimated how much the sleep-deprivation impaired their performance. It can be disastrous not to know what you don't know.

If you're aligned with the latest science tying sleep deprivation to serious health concerns, then you're no longer bragging about *lack* of sleep. Instead, you're bargaining for *sufficient* sleep. Not only is too little sleep detrimental for your brain, it's devastating for your body.

THE STAGES OF SLEEP MATTER

Approximately every ninety minutes, your brain cycles through four stages of sleep: N1, N2, N3, and REM.[4] N1–3 are non-REM stages. The cycles move in this pattern for healthy sleep: N1, N2, N3, N2, REM. About 75 percent of sleep should be in the non-REM stages, with most of that in the N2 phase.

During the N1, N2, and N3 stages tissue repairs itself, new cells grow, and your immune system becomes stronger. Your brain sorts and stabilizes your memories. Stage N3 is particularly integral to better bone, muscle, and immune system health. In REM sleep, your brain sorts through pieces of information to make innovative connections and create solutions. It's also during this stage that your emotions are regulated and reset. Passing properly through these stages of sleep gives you the power to maintain optimism and a good mindset as you work on your health.

WHAT CAUSES POOR SLEEP (EVEN IF YOU'RE NOT SLEEPLESS IN SEATTLE)?

As described earlier, missing even one night of adequate sleep can create physical and mental problems. One of the first things I do when presented with a person in orthopedic pain or interested in wellness or weight loss is to ask about sleep. I am sure that anything else I would prescribe or do would be useless if I can't help with sleep improvement.

THE CIRCADIAN RHYTHM HAS NOTHING TO DO WITH DANCE STEPS

Let's say you go to bed at 10:00 p.m. on Monday night and wake up at 6:00 a.m. Tuesday morning. You might keep this schedule Monday through Friday, and then blow it on the weekends. You might go out to dinner and a movie or go to see a show. You may stay up until midnight and then sleep in until ten. This pushes your bedtime forward by two hours and your waking time forward by four, producing what is known as social jet lag.[5]

We mentioned the importance of circadian rhythm during the discussion in chapter 5 about time-restricted eating. Light stimulates receptors in the eye that connect directly to the brain. Your brain's master control system, the suprachiasmatic nucleus (SCN), sends out daily signals to every other part of your brain and body. This internal circadian rhythm includes physical, mental, and behavioral changes that happen consistently over a twenty-four-hour cycle. Believe it or not, the signals caused by light and dark have dramatic effects on pain levels, stiffness, joint and connective tissue, physical feelings, and mental performance.

Joseph Bass (Northwestern University) has written extensively about the cultural shift that has, in contrast to previous generations, extended our social life and work hours late into the evening. His studies suggest that these changes have disrupted our circadian cycle at the systemic, tissue, and cellular levels. His work also shows how this switch impairs our metabolism and our body as a whole.[6]

Numerous other studies have drawn similar conclusions, suggesting similar levels of misalignment between our circadian rhythm and our choices to sleep and eat at abnormal times—all to the detriment of our health.[7] Personally, I have adopted the social life seen on the television show *The Golden Girls*. I am one of those people eating dinner at five. This allows me to stay within my time-restricted-eating window and my circadian rhythm, yet still participate in life. I am just waiting for everyone else to do it too. I can tell you that my overall pain levels have diminished, and I feel more energetic and stronger throughout the day.

Your physical and mental processes work best when stimuli inside your body and outside in the environment fall into sync.

WHY THE CIRCADIAN RHYTHM MATTERS

If you spend any time listening to wellness podcasts, you are aware of the multitude of therapies available to improve your pain and function. The trouble is that many of these can be time-consuming and expensive. For example, you could buy a hyperbaric chamber, join a health spa, or buy your own sauna and cold-plunge pool. You could use methylene blue suppositories or ozone enemas. You can pay for injections of one substance or another. You could harvest your own blood or stem cells. Even better, you could transfuse a younger person's blood into yourself. A private chef and personal trainer also help.

I practice medicine in the real world. I can assure you that I have never met anyone with the time or money to do such things. Most people are lucky if they can cook often enough to keep the vegetables in the refrigerator from rotting. If you do everything you heard is necessary for your health, there would literally be no time to even say hello to your kids, never mind to be present in their lives.

The most important part of my overall protocol for you is basically cost-free and relatively easy. The first thing you should do to improve your health is to harness a routine. I want you to have a solid routine, each day, with a good sleep-wake cycle and a certain fast-feed window. If you do this and maintain what should be called a constant-routine protocol, you will see benefits in how you feel, and your budget will remain intact. In fact, your budget might even improve.

This probably seems trite right now, but I'll explain how this works. The premise for maintaining a solid schedule comes from recent work in the world of circadian medicine. If you consider the Earth and how we developed on this planet as it orbits the Sun, this will make a lot of sense. Every day, the sun rises and sets. This is based on the Earth's rotation as it orbits the Sun. The circadian rhythm that results from this process is a deeply ingrained, primordial, and universal code to being healthy.[8] Most life on Earth requires this schedule to be respected in order to thrive. For example, plants can only perform photosynthesis during the daytime hours. Some creatures are nocturnal, and their circadian rhythm is flipped from ours, but it is still respected.

A groundbreaking paper in 2012 demonstrated that not only can breaking the circadian rhythm lead to disease but also it can do so without any other inputs. As discussed earlier, it was already well known that feeding an obesogenic diet to mice would induce diabetes and other NCDs. The amazing discovery that followed, however, was that by simply restricting the feeding window, the mice could avoid developing diabetes.[9] Later, the same research group showed that doing the same to metabolically sick mice could cure them.

The connection between respect for daily light-dark oscillations and human health is of immense significance. It is also important that the external cues, such as feeding, match. Miscuing, for example by eating late at night, can throw off the whole rhythm and damage health, including one's joints. When my patients express interest in natural methods to help their bodies feel better, last longer, and become more resilient to stress, I discuss the importance of maintaining a proper routine. I practice a constant routine protocol myself, as does my family. Rarely will I deviate. At first, this was socially awkward since my bedtime is usually around nine, but honestly, no one minds anymore, and they all enjoy our earlier dinner parties. Life is good—and yours can be as well. I have never felt better, and I truly believe that this is due in large part to my better sleep and time-restricted eating. Although I will never achieve perfection, I work to optimize the phase relationship between my central and peripheral clocks. Let me tell you what this has to do with orthopedics and the musculoskeletal system.

Arthritis is just another manifestation of metabolic dysfunction and circadian dysregulation. More and more evidence about osteoarthritis proves it is an inflammatory disease of the entire synovial joint. For my entire medical career, I was led to believe that injury and wear and tear were the only possible reasons that one would develop arthritis. When I learned about things like diet, nutrition, mitochondrial health, chronic inflammation, and oxidative stress, I felt as though a dark lens had been removed from my glasses. Things made much more sense in terms of what I saw in clinical practice. With about 67 percent of Americans overweight or obese, and 88 to 90 percent of us having some kind of metabolic dysfunction (poor mitochondria), you can see why arthritis is so common.

Think of this. We know in orthopedic surgery that most hip and knee arthritis does not happen due to trauma. By contrast, however, we think that most ankle arthritis is due to trauma—indeed, it is thought that up to 80 percent of ankle arthritis is related to a traumatic event. The ankle also bears all of the weight of the body, while the knees and hips do not. That said, ankle arthritis is far less common than hip and knee arthritis. Does this make any sense whatsoever with the injury and wear-and-tear premise?

Cartilage and connective tissue should be flexible yet still capable of supporting weight and movement. During your life, cartilage should be constantly repaired and remodeled. The chondrocytes (cartilage-forming cells) should replace, recycle, and rebuild a degraded extracellular matrix. Generally, this is a slow process in connective tissues as the half-life of collagen-based structures can range from ten years to one hundred years. But the ongoing repair and detoxification of those tissues are what keep us from deteriorating. This requires connective tissues to have the ability to do so. When chondrocytes fail in this function, osteoarthritis happens. This failure is usually due to the same problems that cause other NCDs—chronic low-grade inflammation, oxidative stress, weak mitochondria, and AGE deposition into the tissue. Now, we also understand that a disruption of the circadian rhythm will also dramatically damage the ability of cartilage and connective tissues to repair themselves.

CIRCADIAN RHYTHM AND MUSCULOSKELETAL HEALTH

There is a direct association between inflammation and disease progression of osteoarthritis.[10] Certain cytokine levels are higher with the disease, inducing inflammation and tissue damage. Markers of oxidative stress also increase with osteoarthritis. These molecules compromise function and vitality of your connective tissues at the cellular level. Chondrocytes are reprogrammed into larger cells that are effectively dead—this is called senescence. Basically, this means your chondrocytes become zombie cells, which are never recycled or repaired. Rather, they simply send out more and more damage signals to the immune system to produce further deterioration. The zombie cartilage cells produce proinflammatory cytokines and proteins that degrade the tissue and the extracellular matrix. Mitochondria continue to fail, and your cartilage loses the ability to repair itself. *This* is the real reason for arthritis. Your cartilage is simply unable to do what it is supposed to do in terms of self-repair and restoration.

What does this have to do with your circadian rhythm? Well, cartilage repair, detoxification, restoration, and most other maintenance functions can only happen during sleep, and especially during a fasted sleep. It is important to note that disruption of your circadian clock puts you more at risk for obesity and makes you less able to lose weight.[11] Obesity, as we have discussed, increases levels of chronic low-grade inflammation, and inflammation itself and the immune system in general are also under circadian control. Everything is linked, and everything works better if you stick to a sun-based schedule of sleep and awakening. In order for your body to repair the damage brought about by the stressors of the day, there must be a night. This night must involve good sleep, and you should be fasted. During the night, with elevated levels of melatonin and lower levels of cortisol, repair and restoration of your body can happen. The peripheral clock genes work in a coordinated fashion to achieve this. It cannot happen if you don't sleep well, and it cannot happen if you aren't fasted. You must optimize the feeding and sleep rhythms with those of the light-dark cycle as much as possible. This is key to my protocol for you.

It sounds harder than it is. Basically, you get to sleep. If you then add time-restricted eating to the mix, you don't have to worry so much about how much you eat and, in my opinion, the Mediterranean diet style is the best choice for your window.

There is one caveat to this aspect of the protocol. You cannot decide that going to bed early one evening will produce a dramatic healing event. This process of circadian clock gene optimization takes time to become part of you. Genes must be trained by a solid schedule over time, and so you cannot use a circadian rhythm haphazardly and randomly. This is a lifestyle change—and you must commit. Once you have a constant routine protocol of a solid circadian rhythm, your joints, ligaments, muscle and bone, and all other organs will reap the benefits, and aches and pains will dramatically diminish.

Chapter Seven

SUPPLEMENTS THAT
OFFER SUPPORT

The doctor of the future will no longer treat the human frame with
drugs, but rather will cure and prevent disease with nutrition.
—Thomas Edison, inventor and businessperson

Let's say you're eating good food, exercising properly, sleeping well, and thinking positively. So why might you need supplements?

The typical American diet consists of the following 70 to 80 percent ultra-processed or processed foods.

Type	Monthly	Weekly
Animal protein	22 pounds	5.5 pounds
Added sugars	10.25 pounds	2.56 pounds
Cheese	3.3 pounds	0.83 pounds

It is known that we lose about a decade of life from our diets. If you consider all of the pollution and mental stress in which we exist, you can see how a protocol to improve your health might be needed.

SIGNS THAT SUGGEST YOUR SYSTEM NEEDS A BOOST

Many people catch a cold at least once a year. Some people succumb even more often than that. But if you're constantly catching colds that stick around for weeks or even months, please understand that your immune system is struggling to fight viruses and bacteria.

Fatigue is another sign that you need a boost. Typically feeling tired and strung out even when you haven't been doing anything strenuous? Fatigue flashes yet another warning that your immune system is overworking itself. Even after a good night's sleep, you might still feel exhausted because your body is using all of its energy to fight off viruses and bacteria—even if specific symptoms haven't yet surfaced. When your immune system becomes overwhelmed and can't help your brain to detoxify and repair cells during your sleep, fatigue can be overwhelming. Brain fog might be another subtle sign of a lack of health. Poor mood, irritability, lack of resilience to stress, poor wound healing, and even dry skin can suggest that one's health requires optimization. Other key warning signs are a frequently upset stomach or diarrhea (or both). Beneficial bacteria and microorganisms that live in your gut metabolize foods and manufacture proteins and other molecules used by your immune system as it fights off attacks. Unbalanced gut bacteria, however, can leave you unprotected. A poorly populated gut biome is a poorly functioning gut.

When your microbiome can't absorb enough nutrients from the foods you eat, that can lead to inflammation, which is the fundamental cause of many chronic diseases. Proper nutrition is mandatory for a good immune system.

HERBAL MEDICINE AND SUPPLEMENTS

Eighty percent of the world's population regularly uses herbal treatments. As the popularity of supplements rises in North America and Europe, you may have concerns and questions about adding this holistic approach I advocate for your routine health care. I have my own line of supplements and other natural remedies, so clearly I am a believer.

Until quite recently, the use of plants and herbs to treat pain and illness was necessary. In fact, 118 of the 150 most commonly prescribed drugs in the United States are derived from plants. Historically, herbal medicines and treatments date back thousands of years. In Iraq, archeological studies support these uses as far back as sixty thousand years ago, and in China, at least eight thousand years ago. If you're looking for a *written* document about natural treatments, you can find that thanks to the Sumerians five thousand years ago.[1] Chinese herbal medicine, Arabian herbal medicine, and Ayurvedic medicine (derived from India) are still in common use today—as well as other natural treatments used throughout the world. The Amazon region of Brazil along with South and Central America is the source of numerous natural therapies, medicines, and treatments. If you'd like to read more about the history of specific herbs, spices, and flavorings, check out the five-article series by Louis E. Grivetti.[2]

Roughly 50 percent of the US population takes dietary supplements.[3] And people have plenty of choices; more than eighty thousand supplements are available. My protocol works best with supplements because of all the issues with our food supply and our time deficits. It is really difficult to prepare all of one's meals at home and to eat nine servings of vegetables and fruits each and every day. Supplements can fill some gaps formed by our busy lifestyles.

Warning: Know your source for any supplements you use. Check the manufacturing information and the country of origin. My preference is to use products made in the United States if at all possible. Also, keep in mind that the FDA does not regulate supplements like they do pharmaceuticals, but the FTC, USDA, and the FDA have varying levels of control regarding safety and such, so there is oversight. Use your common sense here; if a supplement is really cheap, it is probably really cheap.

For me, supplements are a mandatory investment for my future health and wellness. They also help me to feel the best I can now and perform at a high level in family life and work.

COST CALCULATIONS—A REAL CONCERN THAT DOESN'T ADD UP

Consumer mindsets have changed—particularly among those who fall into the higher-income and best-educated brackets. For the most part, they've responded favorably to natural treatments and supplements.

Still, the costs of these alternative natural treatments can be of concern to many people—especially during periods of economic downturns. So let's do some real cost comparisons regarding the value of supplements.

First, consider the advantage of staying well versus staying sick. The cost of chemical drugs on your body can be crushing—in both dollars and failing health. Consider the common side effects of nonsteroidal anti-inflammatory drugs, NSAIDs—drugs like ibuprofen, naproxen, diclofenac, celecoxib, mefenamic acid, etoricoxib, indomethacin, and high-dose aspirin. Common side effects of these chemicals include indigestion, stomach ulcers, gastric bleeding, headaches, drowsiness, dizziness. For some people, NSAIDs can even cause serious cardiac side effects.

In addition to considering pain versus good health, for a true cost comparison, consider the true cost of sickness: loss of salary or income while sick and unable to work, the cost of medical visits, your co-pays for medicines, and so forth. The out-of-pocket cost for a severe heart attack in the United States is about $1 million. This includes all the direct costs such as the doctor, the hospital, any medical procedures, diagnostic imaging, and medications. The out-of-pocket costs for a total joint replacement likewise are quite high. It makes financial sense to avoid these eventualities if at all possible.

Congress has given us some cost relief, however, with health savings accounts (HSAs). If your doctor writes a prescription for supplements related to some disease or condition, these items can be paid for out of your HSA. Even if you don't have an HSA set up, you may still be able to deduct the cost of supplements; check with your CPA or tax expert. An HSA is pretax money, and this means that you get a built-in 30 to 50 percent discount on anything that you purchase with it. This is a great vehicle not just to improve your physical health, but also your financial health. These accounts are allowed to roll over year after year if they are not used.

While there's certainly a role for prescription medications, and while you should always check with your personal physician for their recommendations related to your own condition or disease, more than 50 percent of Americans using alternative medicines and treatments insist that their improved health speaks for itself.

SUPPLEMENTS FOR YOUR MEDS CHECKLIST AND MUSCULOSKELETAL HEALTH

In appendix I, I have provided a full list of supplements that I recommend for you. This list includes the ailments that they can treat or prevent, their active ingredients, and information about safe doses, warnings, or overdose potential. Appendix II provides a list of supplements organized by health condition, along with a sample protocol, so that you can easily look up a certain condition and then see how we can use supplements in practice.

It is worth noting that the list includes numerous supplements containing flavonoids, a diverse class of chemical compounds created from plants. They serve a diversity of purposes such as providing pigmentation and UV protection as well as assisting the plant's immune system. You'll find lots of flavonoids in foods you eat every day—in fruits, vegetables, herbs, olive oil, tea, cocoa, wine, soy and fava beans, rice bran, nuts, and vinegars.

Flavonoids are free radical scavengers with strong antioxidant benefits, and as such, they provide relief both from inflammation and from oxidative stress. They also reduce platelet clotting and reduce capillary frailty, therein protecting your cardiovascular system. Flavonoids are also antiaging and anti-allergenic, and promote better mitochondrial function. As discussed earlier, mitochondrial dysfunction is responsible for most of our aches and pains.

If you follow a Mediterranean dietary pattern, you will consume a lot of these chemicals. Supplements merely augment what should be in your meals. When planning meals, think of variety to get all the nutrients you need. If for some reason you cannot eat a balanced diet (or can't eat enough of the right foods), then add supplements as necessary to meet your daily needs.

In determining your daily needs, you may want to access the various government websites for their recommendations. Do keep in mind, however, that these sites state *minimum* daily requirements. They also do not provide dosage recommendations if you hope to prevent, treat, or improve certain conditions or diseases. It is up to you and me to optimize our bodies and brains for maximum function, longevity, and reduced pain.

Always check with your physician before starting a new supplement—particularly one that you intend to continue long term. For instance, many herbs, foods, and dietary supplements can interact significantly with specific anticancer drugs and treatments.[4] You may find that your personal physician or orthopedic surgeon does not have a great depth of knowledge regarding optimal health, wellness, and supplements in particular. This is not their fault; remember that most medical schools don't even bother to teach nutrition. If you feel that your physician cannot answer your questions, you may wish to find second or even third opinions.

Good health and good sense are two
of life's greatest blessings.
—PUBLILIUS SYRUS

Chapter Eight

THERAPIES AND ALTERNATIVE NATURAL TREATMENTS

The art of medicine consists of amusing the patient while nature cures the disease.

—Voltaire

We humans are an impatient lot. We're used to having our dry cleaning done in an hour, pizza delivery in half an hour, and a website loaded in fewer than three seconds. Instant gratification is expected, and many of us can become angry if there is any sort of delay, no matter what the product or service.

When it comes to health care, we expect the same speed: Swallow a pill and feel better in four hours. Undergo a joint replacement in the morning and leave the hospital later the same day. But with natural, noninvasive treatments, we may wait two to three months to see results—without the risks of surgeries and the cost and inconvenience of lifetime pharmaceuticals to maintain the status quo. One of my greatest struggles with my own patients is to convince them to give natural remedies, diet, and nutrition a proper chance. When and if they do, the changes can be remarkable. By writing this book, I hope that I have provided an avenue of explanation for a world with no time.

Because of the medical-food-pharmaceutical-insurance complex, we've been led to believe that poor health is inevitable and only medications to modify a cell, an enzyme, or a hormone can possibly heal us. What's more, governmental regulatory agencies have blessed that concept. It is often said there are no "good" studies on natural methods of healing, such as improved diet, supplements, exercise, and the like. This is because these studies are hard to do, and frankly, there is not a lot of money to fund them because you can't patent and sell the methods. However, I have told you about all of the work done on the Mediterranean diet and how successful it can be in reducing pain, arthritis, and improving overall health.

Recently, I completed an evaluation for the Department of Veterans Affairs concerning a patient's disability claim. The patient had deployed as a Marine in 2003, 2004, and 2005. He suffered back pain, headaches, and a traumatic brain injury (TBI) from a roadside bomb during one deployment, and then a rocket attack during another. According to the paperwork attached to the disability claim, it took this patient more than five years to get his claim approved. Why so long? Agency reps kept denying it because there were no records of the patient taking pain medications. The Marine had refused to take narcotics. It took him the first three years to find a physician willing to work with him rather than just write a prescription for painkillers. With that physician's treatment plan, he now uses deep diaphragmatic breathing, mindfulness, and meditation to treat his symptoms and control his pain.

I share this example of how difficult it is for people who really want to avoid surgery and narcotics and instead be healthy for life, despite any given injury or problem. There is no incentive to treat anything or anyone naturally using lifestyle and dietary changes. Rather, the benefits are geared toward those who take pharmaceuticals, have surgery, and fail treatments, all the while never overcoming their impairments. This does not bode well for a "life well lived" in most cases. I think we can do better as a society.

Proper food can become a healing medicine. Restorative sleep repairs our cells. Following a set schedule that mirrors the revolutions of the earth and sun triggers immense cellular benefits. Exercise invigorates us. And a positive mindset helps control pain and improve function of both body and mind. That's not to say lifestyle changes are easy—they aren't.

But why don't we at least hear about these natural options more often from physicians? The obvious answer: Most physicians receive little or no training in natural treatments, exercise, or nutrition, so these choices never come to their minds. Likewise, how is it possible to explain all of this in a single office visit?

Surgery and medications serve as a quick fix, but often simply delay getting to the root of a health problem and correcting it for long-term wellness. These quick fixes can even become addictive and dangerous. Of course, sometimes surgery and pharmaceuticals are required. However, following this healthy life protocol will make such treatments even more effective for you. By combining all-natural treatments and conventional medicine—the best methods and treatments from both philosophies—patient outcomes can be optimized. I practice medicine this way.

In earlier chapters, we've highlighted evidence that shows surgical outcomes are often no better than natural treatments—or even doing nothing at all. Surgery presents more risks including infections, adverse reactions to anesthesia, complications in healing, and reoccurrence of the original problem(s). Surgery is often indicated in the false biomedical "abnormality" thesis. Surgery is, of course, a covered service, and wellness is not.

In longer-term studies where the researchers gave sufficient time for natural treatments to work, the outcomes after natural treatments matched surgery outcomes—but without many of the risks. There are few orthopedic studies that mention sleep schedule, stress level, diet pattern, and exercise protocol of the subjects. Occasionally one or two variables regarding lifestyle are examined, but not usually. There is definitely never a mention of alternative methods to heal.

It's important to state at the outset that one of your biggest impediments to natural treatments for orthopedic conditions, aches and pains, stiffness, and such issues will be coverage. The *Journal of the American Medical Association* actually looked at insurance coverage from 2010 to 2019 and found that coverage was sporadic. Even when it was covered, the insurance companies forced a higher copay or coinsurance.

*The way you think, the way you behave, the way
you eat, can influence your life by 30 to 50 years.*
—DEEPAK CHOPRA

THE POWER OF THE SUN TO TREAT PAIN AND IMPROVE YOUR HEALTH

For too long, we have ignored the skin, yet this organ provides the largest surface area for treatment. The skin also serves as a conduit for fluids, minerals, heat, and toxins. The skin has vast interconnections with the brain, the nervous system, and other physiologic systems of the body.

Skin has a neuroectodermal origin, meaning that it shares features with the nervous system. Positive changes related to your pain happen when photons of the sun interact with your skin and eyes.

Like all stressors available to us, UVB (ultraviolet radiation)—part of the energy delivered by the sun—is a double-edged sword. UVB can cause cancer (and wrinkles), but it also helps reduce pain and coordinate cortisol with melatonin to manage your circadian rhythm. UVB also stimulates the melanin pigment and helps to make vitamin D3. UVB coordination between the skin and brain can also suppress an overly aggressive immune system. In fact, UVB exposure is one of the primary treatments for psoriasis.

There's a lot of give-and-take between the skin and the brain, and between the immune system and the endocrine system.

Ample Vitamin D3

Studies show a strong link between vitamin D3 levels and pain—back pain, arthritic pain, and widespread chronic pain. Sunlight exposure and vitamin D3 supplements also lead to better sleep. Better sleep leads to less pain and fewer pathologic musculoskeletal conditions. More vitamin D3 also leads to a lower incidence of depression—and less depression leads to less pain.

As you can see, these three things set up a chain reaction: Without ample sunlight, vitamin D3, and sleep, you feel more pain. Having ample sunlight, vitamin D3, and sleep leads to less pain. Each of these three factors are interdependent.

In a study of eighty-nine patients conducted in 2005, researcher J. M. Walch and his team demonstrated the effects of sunlight on pain medication. After spine surgery, patients were placed in either a bright or dim hospital room. The brighter rooms had about 46 percent more natural sunlight, and those in the bright rooms used 22 percent fewer opioid medications for their pain. In addition, patients in the bright rooms reported less stress and had fewer complaints of pain.

Another study showed that bright hospital rooms led to shorter hospital stays after heart surgery. More importantly, this study also showed that there were fewer deaths among patients in brighter rooms. One explanation is that light exposure increases serotonin in the body.

Light exposure is a valid way to improve mood. We know that an improved mood and mindset lead to less pain and better function. In fact, light treatment for depression can be as good as medicine, and with far with fewer side effects. So one simple way to decrease your pain would be to sit by a window every day; better, sit outside for about thirty minutes instead.

Both sunlight exposure and high serum levels of vitamin D are associated with less cartilage loss in the knee. A deficiency of vitamin D is strongly linked to subchondral bone fractures and swelling (fractures below the cartilage on the weight-bearing surface of a bone).

Of course, the photobiomodulation of pain does not happen simply because of vitamin D. There is a complex interplay between light-sensing retinal structures and areas of the brain responsible for pain. These areas are integral to pain modification.

HOW TO STOP THE PAIN

As we have discussed throughout, there are many issues that affect how, why, or when we feel pain. Now, let's focus on putting a stop to that pain with some additional methods. I often find myself recommending a nice trip to the beach for patients that need overall wellness therapy. Not only does walking in sand provide excellent rehabilitation for certain foot, ankle, knee, hip, and spine problems, but something about the beach just feels great. There is a reason that health resorts are often located in sunny and beachy areas. Restoration is not happening simply because of time off and relaxation; after all, there are no resorts in caves, right? There is something about nature, sunlight, and fresh air that is extremely healthy. People have known this forever, but only now can we delineate the scientific mechanisms that account for the healing power of nature.

Exposure to Green Spaces

Being in nature—for example, walking on paths that weave through trees and plants—means that we will be exposed to sunlight. Even on a cloudy or rainy day, we have sunlight. It is well known that being in nature is relaxing and can reduce stress, anxiety, and pain. Numerous studies have shown that this combination of green spaces and sunlight exposure reduces our stress and improves our mental health.

While you're out in nature soaking up the sunlight, here's what's going on inside your body: The sunlight exposure leads to the production of melatonin (eventually), beta-endorphin (a natural pain killer), and nitric oxide (a vasodilator that dilates your blood vessels). Without the initial spike of cortisol early in the day, the later spike of melatonin and good sleep are not possible. In addition, we know that sunlight induces the expression of the POMC gene, which leads to cortisol production and more beta-endorphins.

In a recent review of nature-based-therapies, two theories were discussed. These were the stress reduction theory (SRT) of Roger Ulrich and the attention restoration theory (ART) of Rachel and Stephen Kaplan. The review concluded that "contact with nature can decrease psychological and physiological stress, restore cognitive focus, and increase feelings of relaxation."

Photobiomodulation: Light Therapy

Parents who've had a baby born with a slightly yellow skin understand the power of phototherapy. UV light is very successful at treating jaundice in newborns. The pediatrician places a blindfold on the infant to protect the eyes and places the baby in an incubator under bright lights. Voilà! In a few days, the yellow skin turns to a natural pigment. Evidence is growing that photobiomodulation therapy—PBM therapy—works very well for a variety of other conditions.

This therapy varies slightly because light itself varies with different wavelengths, intensities, and applications. If you apply a certain wavelength of light to different parts of the body, you'll get different results. For example, the same wavelength of light in the red spectrum can help reduce neuropathy pain and migraine-headache pain. But the light is applied differently. To reduce neuropathy pain, the light penetrates through the skin. By contrast, to reduce pain from migraines, the light is applied through the retina. Blue light seems to cause pain in some people with migraines, while green light reduces that pain. This is because green light seems to cause the formation of natural pain killers. Studies of the spinal cord of rats exposed to green light found increased proenkephalin-A mRNA. This enkephalin is a natural pain killer that our bodies make every day. So basically, the green light inhibits pain signals.[1]

Green light also plays a role in the body's response to potentially toxic stimuli like chemicals, injuries, or adverse temperatures. Green light is particularly useful when delivering light treatment through the eyes, versus through the skin.

Dim light at night will disturb sleep by reducing melatonin production in your body.[2] You'll also recall that disruptions in the daily sleep pattern increase pain, as shown in studies of night-shift workers. More specifically, pain from neuroinflammation is caused by exposure to light while sleeping. Additionally, if red light is applied visually, pain increases; but the opposite is true if red light is applied through the skin.[3]

The skin serves as another route through which we might reduce aches and pains with photons. Direct contact of 950 nm infrared light on incision sites can reduce sensitivity. Infrared light administered to an incision site will also reduce dilation of your blood vessels from nitric oxide, reducing the inflammation and pain. The same wavelength of light applied to the skin also reduces inflammation and oxidative stress causing pain.[4]

LED Light versus Laser Light

The color, the wavelength, and the delivery method all matter for effectiveness of photobiomodulation and the specific area of the body that you're treating.

With LASER—light amplification by stimulated emission of radiation—there's a greater risk of thermal injury than with LED lights. That's because with a laser, the light is monochromatic and 100 percent coherent. In other words, it's a strong beam of light synchronized in space and time. By contrast, LED light is not monochromatic and is noncoherent, and involves a narrow range of light. So LED is safer, but it also delivers less energy.

The shorter wavelengths of light work better delivered through the visual system and the opsin cells in the eye. So, as mentioned earlier, green light is used for this purpose. These cone-driven signals lead to less pain. However, the treatment durations are much longer—hours versus minutes—for the shorter wavelengths than for the longer ones.[5]

The body's response to bright light and sunlight depends on changes that happen in the brain. Once stimulated, the visual circuit sends signals to certain areas of the brain. This process essentially suppresses your perception of pain. In other words, bright light can alter the pain signals so that your brain does not feel as much.[6] And this is excellent news for a great many people—those with pain after surgery and those with headaches, fibromyalgia, arthritis, and low-back pain.

Laser therapy (also known as LLLT, low-level laser therapy) has been used for osteoarthritis for nearly thirty years. This laser therapy comes from pure light of a single wavelength and works by causing photochemical reactions in cells. Patients with rheumatoid arthritis treated with laser therapy had a 70 percent reduction in pain, as compared to the control group. They also experienced significant improvements in stiffness and flexibility in their hands.[7]

A Balancing Act Between Light and Proper Hormone Levels

Finally, another way that sunlight reduces our sense of pain and unhappiness is by helping us maintain proper hormone levels. UVB exposure to the skin increases our levels of the sex-steroid hormones. To get specific, the skin's exposure to the sun improves the function of the hypothalamic-pituitary-adrenal axis, the gonadal axis, and the resulting hormone levels. For example, testosterone generally increases with sunlight exposure, reducing our perception of pain.

So now you know why you feel better after a trip to the beach—greater exposure to the sun through the skin and eyes. Obviously, you should protect yourself from skin cancer, but avoiding the sun altogether can be just as harmful as too much sun. As with much of life, you need to find a balance.

HOT AND COLD

The power of heat and cold cannot be overstated. Thermal stressors can reduce pain by reducing inflammation, oxidative stress, removing toxins, and increasing resiliency. Plus, exposing your body to uncomfortable temperatures turns on your longevity genes to slow the natural aging process.

In other words, when you work, play, and live in similar temperatures year-round, your body doesn't have to work very hard to stay comfortable. But everything changes when you put yourself in uncomfortable temperatures. When your body has to work hard to stay warm or cool, good things happen inside. Your breathing rate has to adapt. Your heart rate has to either slow down or speed up. Your blood flow throughout the skin, your largest organ, changes to accommodate the extreme temperatures you're exposing yourself to during either cold or heat treatment. All that's good, purposeful, healing.

Basically, what's happening inside your body with a temperature change follows a fundamental biological principle: homeostasis, the tendency for all living things to try to maintain stability in all systems. As it relates to heat and cold treatment, if your body gets too hot, the homeostasis process cools you down. Likewise, if your body gets too cold, the homeostasis process warms you up. A very hot external environment will result in a cool core. A very cold external environment will result in a warm core. Thermal stress does even more to improve your physiology.

Let's discuss heat treatments first, then cold.

So You Say You Want a Sauna?

Traditionally, when we think of saunas, we picture an exclusive resort on some exotic island offering sauna bathing at prices that make your head spin. Keep that image in the back of your mind—you'll need it when you start to plan your next vacation.

Using saunas for healing is nothing new. For thousands of years, both dry and wet sauna treatments have been used safely and effectively for healing and long-term good health: Native American sweat lodges. Finnish saunas, dry or steam. Japanese hot baths. Russian *banyas*.

Saunas are particularly effective at reducing pain and lowering the risk of death. Indeed, a review of *dozens of studies* on sauna use shows that consistent sauna sessions can:

- Reduce the risk of cardiovascular disease by 50 percent (lower blood pressure, reduce arterial stiffness, make beneficial changes in lipid profiles, modulate the autonomic nervous system)

- Reduce the risk of Alzheimer's disease by 65 percent (improving blood flow to the brain and lower inflammation in the brain)
- Reduce the risk "significantly" of new onset stroke
- Reduce the risk and severity of depression
- Reduce the risk of pulmonary conditions and diseases (such as pneumonia, colds, flu) by 27 percent
- Improve conditions such as arthritis and headache
- Improve endurance and performance (strength, muscle mass maintenance, cell renewal and growth, joint function)
- Prevent degenerative disease (reduce inflammation)
- Prevent metabolic disease (diabetes and obesity)
- Stimulate the immune system and prevent immunological/autoimmune diseases
- Maintain muscle mass

As we know, Americans are not typically known for patience. Natural treatments like saunas can take up to two or three months to deliver positive outcomes. But if you sincerely want to improve your health without surgeries and meds, patience pays off big time.

Sauna works the same way that exercise, fasting, and cold therapy does; it stresses the body temporarily and allows the cellular stress-response system to engage. Misfolded proteins, mutated DNA, damaged cell membranes, and dysfunctional mitochondria are cleared out and recycled for parts if possible. Stronger and better cell structures result. This is not possible without a stress to the system. Sauna use extends your health span and makes you feel better in the immediate term. Stretching in the sauna is very beneficial to the connective tissues as their compliance increases in high heat. Joint stiffness is decreased in sauna. Likewise, muscle spasm and ischemia is reduced.

In addition, sweating in the sauna is one of the best ways to rid your body of toxic heavy metals. Petrochemicals, heavy metals, and other toxins tend to accumulate in adipose and connective tissues; eliminating these from the body can only help.

Cautions when Considering Sauna Sessions

Despite the abundant evidence for the health benefits of the sauna, it's essential to be careful. In particular, consider the following:

- Assess any ongoing health challenges. Don't use a sauna if you've had a recent heart attack or stroke, have severe aortic stenosis, or have a blocked aorta.
- Don't use a sauna if you have a condition that prevents you from sweating.
- Don't use a sauna if you have certain autoimmune disorders (such as lupus or MS). Raising core body temperature with these conditions is not helpful.
- Don't use a sauna without consulting your physician if you are taking any medication that alters your blood pressure.
- Never get in a sauna while drinking alcohol.
- Consult your own doctor for the recommended number of sessions per week, length of time in a sauna, and the appropriate temperature ranges.
- Stay hydrated. You may lose a pound of fluid per sauna session—as well as losing sodium, chloride, potassium, magnesium, and calcium. When dehydrated you often feel fatigued and may get muscle cramps. So make sure to drink enough fluids to replace lost electrolytes. About sixteen ounces of water per session is the minimum.

Now Let's Discuss Cold

Earlier, we explained how heat and cold therapies basically work on the same stressor principle—but with a different stressor (heat versus cold). Cold will do different things for you than does heat, but both provide thermal stress. As I'm sure you know, cold packs are often used for things like sports injuries. They are effective at decreasing blood circulation, metabolic activity, muscle spasms or cramping, as well as reducing inflammation, swelling, and pain. Cold packs, coolant spray, or gel can be applied two or three times per day (or even once per hour if necessary), for about twenty or thirty minutes per time. It is best to have a thin layer of material between the skin and the source of cold in order to protect the outer layer of skin. Alternating between cold and hot treatment can also provide excellent results. And remember: if you don't have a cold pack, you can make your own by mixing 70 percent rubbing alcohol with water in a sealable plastic bag and freezing it. Now, let's take a look at some other applications for cold treatment.

Cold Immersion

If you listen to any wellness podcasts or read any fitness or antiaging blogs, you probably already know what cold immersion is. Due to the high density of cold receptors in the skin, cold immersion sends an overwhelming number of electrical impulses from peripheral nerve endings to the brain, often resulting in an antidepressive effect.

Cold exposure has myriad benefits for humans that include improved glucose metabolism, reduced inflammation, better immune cell function, and better cognition. It enhances resilience and mood, and allows for less pain. Allow me to briefly explain why I think this should be a part of your overall protocol to preserve and improve your body and brain for a long and happy life. Again, this should only be considered after a discussion with your personal physician.

There are different ways to achieve cold exposure, but the most studied is whole body immersion—that is, up to the neck. Generally, cold is considered to be 59 degrees Fahrenheit or colder. The level of coldness can vary based on your personal tolerance and other factors.

Like fasting, sauna, and exercise, cold exposure utilizes the scientific principle of hormesis. Hormesis is a dose-dependent response to a stressful agent. That is, at low doses, the agent will give benefit, but at high doses, it is toxic. Habitual exposure to cold by intent is helpful. Norepinephrine is released in high levels with immersion in cold water. Likewise, dopamine levels rise dramatically and remain high for hours, and so cold exposure is also known to help with symptoms of depression and anxiety.

Better and healthier mitochondria in your muscle tissue also result after immersion, while cold exposure can also help with glucose levels, since your brown fat—metabolically active fat—takes up more glucose during cold exposure than muscle.

Cold exposure will also cause the release of cold-shock proteins, which, like HSPs, will improve cell survival and help to regenerate damaged neurons. It is also apparent that levels of natural antioxidants increase with cold exposure. Inflammation is reduced with cold, and this helps with the regular aches and pains we associate with orthopedic conditions like arthritis.[8]

The more we see health as a practice rather than as a problem to fix, the more we encourage the body's natural potential to be healthy.
—AARTI PATEL, AMERICAN
PSYCHIATRIST AND AUTHOR

ACUPUNCTURE

Originating in ancient China, this procedure involves pricking the skin or tissues with hair-thin needles at precise points on the body. The practitioner then guides the needles (which may or may not be heated) with specific movements. By stimulating certain points of the body, different treatment effects can be achieved. One of the primary reasons to use acupuncture therapy is to relieve pain, particularly nerve-based and arthritic or muscle pain. The objectives of the treatment might also include alleviating various physical, mental, or emotional conditions.

Practitioners believe that energy meridians pass through all parts of the body and reflect a person's health. A meridian is the path through which *qi*, or vital energy, flows. Their objective is to stimulate the external part of the body (for example, an ear or a wrist) to redirect negative energy from the internal body part that's ill or in pain. Acupuncture works by harnessing the ascending and descending connections between the peripheral and central nervous systems. The needle will stimulate certain peripheral nerves that will then either enhance or diminish pain signals along the same track. The tracks of communications seem to mimic the meridian maps.

Because acupuncture treatments are invasive—even if only mildly—some patients experience side effects for a few days, like nausea, skin rashes, dizziness, pain, bruising, bleeding, or infections from the needle pricks. It is important to find a well-trained practitioner if you wish to add this modality to your personal health protocol. Some physicians believe the effects of acupuncture may be from placebo effects only. However, pain relief and improved function are real effects even if due from a mindset adjustment, placebo effect, or a "true" (medical) treatment effect. I have seen acupuncture do wonders for my patients, and I think it should be considered by anyone interested in avoiding synthetic drugs, steroid injections, or surgery.

Studies addressing the efficacy of acupuncture offer encouraging results. For instance, one study looking at people with rheumatoid arthritis found that acupuncture helped them with pain, and suggested that it should be available as an adjunctive care.[9] A recent review of multiple studies of acupuncture for knee osteoarthritis found that it was beneficial both for pain relief and also for improving function along with quality of life.[10] I have found myself recommending acupuncture for my fibromyalgia patients as well. There is good evidence that it is beneficial for this widespread pain syndrome too.

Discuss any planned acupuncture treatments with your doctor, and hopefully, you have some insurance coverage. If you do not, maybe you will be able to utilize an HSA, HRA, or flex account. For a list of acupuncturists in your local area, check with the American Academy of Medical Acupuncture at www.medicalacupuncture.org.

PHYSICAL THERAPY

A primary part of my ability to treat and heal orthopedic conditions nonoperatively is because of my team of physical therapists. I designed my office so that the PT gym would be smack in the middle of my office building, meaning that I am able to work very closely with the therapists in designing protocols based on the precise individual needs of the patients. My surgical schedule is much lighter because of the power of physical therapy to make many problems better.

There are very complicated connections between lines of fascia in the body and various joints and muscles. By employing different techniques, a therapist can use these connections to improve things. For example, the lateral (outside) ankle is connected to the pubis by way of interconnected fascial lines that wrap around the foot and move up the inside of the leg. There is another line that connects the plantar fascia to the skull. If you want to see this in action, do the following (if able): stand with feet flat and try to touch the floor with your fingers. If you can't, roll the bottom of your feet on tennis balls for five minutes or so. Try again. The second try will be much more successful because the plantar fascia deep-tissue work allowed a release of that fascial line that runs up the back to the skull.

I could go on and on about the wonders of PT, but that would fill another couple of books. If your physician does not believe in the power of the human body and the wonderful profession of physical therapy, see if you have direct access in your state. Many states now allow patients to seek care of physical therapists without a prescription. Full disclosure, I was the only physician in the State of Louisiana to advocate for direct access for the people of this state when the bill came before our legislature. I have also been appointed by our governor to sit on the Board of Physical Therapy. Obviously, I am a strong proponent of this vital part of orthopedic care.

The idea is to die young as late as possible.
—ASHLEY MONTAGU, BRITISH-
AMERICAN ANTHROPOLOGIST

Although we've come to the end of the chapter, we're definitely not to the end of natural treatments that can reduce pain and restore health. New natural treatments will surface every year. Make it your goal to stay abreast of the latest natural remedies to avoid unnecessary surgery, invasive procedures, and the harmful side effects of medicines. I have focused on a few main adjunctive modalities that you can use to help avoid surgery or to make your outcomes better. These have a lot of studies and evidence behind them. However, just because a natural method does not have a lot of studies does not mean it is not safe, effective, or worth trying. Rather, that just means that a scientist did not receive funding to do the work.

What have you got to gain? Pain-free living!

Chapter Nine

CUE UP QUESTIONS TO ASK YOUR DOCTOR

The art of medicine consists of amusing the patient while nature cures the disease.

—Voltaire, French author and philosopher

During technical writing workshops for Fortune 500 organizations, the participants—attorneys, engineers, medical experts, or systems analysts—frequently push back when we suggest they write procedures or reports in plain English.

Their rallying cry: "But everybody understands this jargon!"

No, they don't.

The workshop facilitator shows how "everybody" fails to understand by asking participants to pass their gobbledygook to a colleague who will state their conclusions after reading it. The results are both revealing and amusing. So to those students, the facilitator quotes Albert Einstein: "If you can't explain it simply, you don't understand it well enough."

And that applies equally to doctors. If your doctor can't explain the diagnosis and recommended treatment in terms you can understand, the doctor either (1) doesn't understand what the scans, the numbers, and the tests reveal, or (2) they may lack the communication skills to be in practice.

The late Charlie T. (Tremendous) Jones, a motivational speaker, was known around the world for this motto: "You'll be the same five years from now as you are today—except for the books you read and the people you meet." Our twist on that motto: "You'll be in the same unhealthy condition five years from now as you are now—except for the Warner Well Theory MEDS, the doctors you see, and the books you read."

What that means basically is taking control of your health care—knowing what works and what doesn't. Research. Ask questions. Understand your test results. Make informed, smart decisions about how to live well and long.

But that advice doesn't mean all doctors will be thrilled about your research. Gladys is a case in point.

Gladys could be characterized as spunky for her age (ninety-two). Having been in the workforce for more years than she cared to count, she'd grown independent and skeptical of anyone trying to sell her on a product or service. And that came to be her family doctor—the salesperson for semiannual visits and unnecessary tests.

On a recent visit to her doctor, he explained because of how Medicare "set up the system," she needed to come see him twice a year and have whatever tests he deemed necessary. He went on to explain that Medicare didn't reimburse him enough for these office visits, and he couldn't afford to keep her as a patient if she didn't comply with his testing recommendations—that those test charges "made up the difference" financially for him.

So she complied for years, coming in as scheduled for the semiannual visits and various tests. But finally, on one of those visits, she decided to revolt against the prescribed test. When the doctor told her that her kidney function was failing and she needed to undergo more tests, she pointed out that she had gone to the ER recently due to high blood pressure, where she was admitted for observation, and they ran similar tests.

The hospital test results proved to be in the acceptable range. All was well, according to the hospitalist, who dismissed her without medications or further instructions.

But then back to her family doctor and his recommendations for more tests, Gladys pointed out she'd completed all her "recommended" tests and wasn't willing to undergo more.

Gladys was quite agitated and was no longer compliant. Her family doctor walked her back to the lobby area, handed her chart to the receptionist for refiling, and told Gladys that he could no longer see her. No reason given. Shortly afterward, Gladys received an official letter of dismissal, telling her that she had thirty days to find another family physician.

So she did.

And her new doctor saw no reason at all for the earlier "recommended" tests. Now at age ninety-seven, she's still in good health and still takes doctor's "orders" with the proverbial grain of salt since she "knows her own body."

Good for Gladys. When you're in a similar situation, at the least, get a second opinion about a serious diagnosis and the recommended treatment. On the other hand, most doctors do not order enough tests or the right tests in my opinion. Certainly, the average orthopedic surgeon is not considering the true underlying reason for a patients' aches and pains. I do, however—and I am going to give you a list of what you should look for in your personal bloodwork.

An astounding, compelling study published a few years ago analyzed the medical records of 286 patients referred to the Mayo Clinic for second opinions. The conclusion: the first and second opinions were the same in only 12 percent of these 286 situations.[1]

The seemingly obvious point: Doctors make mistakes. They are not infallible. Often, mistakes result from the fact that they typically spend only five to ten minutes per visit talking with their patients about their symptoms. It's likely that your own experience bears this out. Doctors can engage in groupthink, and usually only do what their group, hospital, or neighbor is doing. Think-ing outside of the box is often discouraged in medicine. Another issue is that doctors learn only the recommended daily allowances, do not learn any real nutrition knowledge, and are not taught the true reason for chronic diseases like arthritis, not to mention heart disease, diabetes, cancer, dementia, and the like.

It would seem that you are responsible for your own health and wellness. Consider the case of Consuela, diagnosed with cancer:

As a busy management consultant, Consuela (a vivacious sixty-year-old) understands the importance of second opinions. In fact, that's why con-sultants such as herself get hired by major corporations—to offer outside opinions and expert recommendations that internal management overlooks because of their blind spots.

So when her long-time ob-gyn found a lump in her breast (which a biopsy showed to be malignant) and referred her to an oncologist, she visited the oncologist about treatment. But in the back of her mind, she knew she would not stop with that one oncology visit. Used to educating herself in her role as an external consultant, she began her breast-cancer education process by getting a second and third opinion and by reading massive numbers of health-care journal articles and books on the topic.

While the doctors told her she had only one viable option (surgery, mas-tectomy, plastic surgery), she refused to accept that treatment course without comprehensive research about her cancer and potential treatments.

Her conclusion? The most profitable procedure for hospitals and other health-care professionals is chemotherapy. The more cases and controversial studies she reviewed, the more skeptical she became that the "only" treat-ment, if she wanted to live, was the conventional path of surgery, chemo, and radiation. Even her family members pleaded for her to "just go along" with the doctor.

Despite the lack of encouragement from the health-care profession-als and family, Consuela opted for natural treatments. She contacted a nutritionist in the Chicago area for diet plans, hired an exercise therapist, and started supplements.

Two years later, the lump (which she calls Sadie) is still in her breast. But she insists she feels better than she's ever felt in her life on her self-prescribed regimen.

Of course, no one knows the final outcome with Consuela, but she's happy with her choices now and living life to the fullest—and still traveling the world and putting in long hours as a management consultant

Now I know a fair number of cancer surgeons and plastic surgeons, and sometimes removal of a tumor is absolutely the best choice. What would be awesome though is if your body would fight off the cancer nidus prior to growth into a tumor. That is where the lifestyle I am asking you to live comes into play.

While cancer is potentially more complex than aches and pains, to live your best life without creaky joints, you need this protocol. If you follow this life, I bet your overall health improves dramatically, to include any mood disorders. Watch as your biomarkers improve and know that not only are you ridding your body of weakness and pain, but you are also reducing your risk of major chronic disease.

Concierge care, of course, promises more attention—but not necessarily different thinking. That is, many doctors create new plans, whereby the patient pays a set annual fee (like a retainer) and is not charged visit by visit. As a plus to this plan, the physician becomes available to the patient twenty-four/seven by phone or text for questions, to prescribe medications, or to run tests. Although many patients love these concierge services with the extra attention and prompt responses, they say they're still getting the same conventional treatments.

The medical field resembles any other field—high tech, engineering, defense. Professionals must stay up to date with the latest science and technology. No matter how caring or compassionate your doctor may be, above all, they should offer quality care. That said, most physicians are completely boxed in by the hospitals that employ them or by the insurance companies' policies for coverage.

If you want to investigate more natural ways of living long and well, you may find it necessary to branch out on your own with self-education. Or find a good health consultant. I have become such a consultant to assist in the management of optimal health. It is important for you to understand there is standard health and optimal health. We want to be optimal. At the very least, we hope that this chapter—and, indeed, this book—will prompt you to ask the right questions of your doctors.

What follow here are questions about various tests and diagnostic bio-markers that can lead you to discover potential problems down the line, so you can take preventative measures. Ignorance is not bliss; it's downright dangerous and leads to preventable aches and pain, disease, and early death.

Standard medicine will ask you to only achieve standard results of standard lab tests. One thing you should know about "normal" ranges in blood work is that the normal is based on the population. So, if the population is 50 to 60 percent obese and 90 percent metabolically deranged, then the "normal" ranges are not going to be optimal for you and me. Likewise, the recommended daily allowance (RDA) for nutrients was first developed during World War II. The point of the RDA was to increase survival rates of soldiers. The RDA was designed to achieve the bare minimum for prevention of deficiency disease, but it is not set up for optimal health. For D3 levels, for instance, I want a level of fifty to eighty. The normal range is set at greater than or equal to thirty. The normal range ensures there will not be rickets—but it is not optimal.

So if you are shooting for normal ranges of micronutrients and basing your intake of them on the RDA, you probably won't get scurvy, rickets, pellagra, beriberi, or other deficiency diseases. But you certainly won't live the best life possible either. The last update to the RDA was in 1997, and it was based on average body weights. Bear in mind, back then, the average woman weighed 135 pounds—today she is 170 pounds. Back then, the average weight for a man was 166 pounds, and today it is closer to 200 pounds. So, this would make even the bare minimum of the RDA perhaps inadequate.

Likewise, know that most ranges that are considered "normal" when you get your regular blood work are based on the American population. What is normal has changed over time as our country has become sicker. For example, the "normal" levels of AST and ALT (liver biomarkers) have increased over the past decades as fatty liver has become more and more common.

I want you to understand your overall health and your lab work because it really matters for your joints, muscle, connective tissues, skin, and so on. It matters not just for your brain and cardiovascular health, but also for how your body feels now. If your numbers are not optimal, you are at risk of being indicated for orthopedic surgery. I realize that you are not likely to be asked about your metabolic health at a standard orthopedic clinic visit, but in my opinion, that is the core issue, and it should be handled. My goal for you is to get your house in order and avoid any potential orthopedic surgeries. This may not be possible for some, depending on the diagnosis, but if these biomarkers are improved, so will be the surgical outcomes.

GENERAL QUESTIONS FOR MOST ANY DOCTOR VISIT

Keep these questions on a checklist to carry with you to doctor visits when contemplating an orthopedic procedure.

- Why are we doing the X test or MRI? Will this change the management of my problem?
- What will the X test or MRI show?
- What is the data on the asymptomatic population undergoing the same MRI?
- Is it possible any of my current medications or supplements are causing or complicating this condition?
- Do you see any negative interactions between my medications, supplements, or over-the-counter medicines?
- What are the potential risks or side effects of this procedure/surgery?
- How much function will I gain from this procedure realistically?
- Is your recommended treatment aimed at controlling symptoms or as a cure for the problem?

- What's the success rate (track record) of this procedure/surgery for people in my condition?
- What can I expect during recovery—and how long will the typical recovery take?
- How specifically can I expect to improve after the treatment/surgery? Are there symptoms that will not improve even after treatment?
- How long will your recommended treatment last? Will I have to have a redo at some later point?
- Is your recommended treatment the typical one nationally for my condition?
- Other than what you're recommending, what other options do I have to resolve this issue/problem?
- What natural treatments or therapies might accomplish the same positive outcome?
- What likely happens to me if I do nothing to treat this condition?
- Can you give me some names of colleagues to give a second opinion?

Those are, I think, basic questions. However, what you should really be asking is "Why do I have arthritis or tendinitis or pain?" If the answer is "because you are old" or "because you are obese," maybe consider another opinion elsewhere. True, age and obesity are the most common risk factors for arthritis and other chronic diseases, but the fundamental problem is with the cellular function of the mitochondria and with insulin resistance. It takes a number of decades to destroy the mitochondria and your ability to use insulin, so thus, age. Obesity is the canary in the coal mine for metabolic disease, including metabolic disease of the joints, so thus, obesity.

You need to know if you are insulin resistant, if you have fatty liver, if you are inflamed and if you are deficient in micronutrients. This is the least you should be allowed to know about yourself. I will warn you, most of this may end up being a cash outlay for you because your insurance company does not agree with me.

As I told you, almost 90 percent of this country is metabolically deranged. The National Institutes of Health define this syndrome as having three of these five issues:

- A waist that is ≥35 inches for women, or ≥40 inches for men
- Blood pressure of 130/85mm/Hg
- Reduced HDL with levels of ≤40 mg/dL
- High triglyceride levels of ≥150 mg/dL
- Fasting blood glucose of ≥100 mg/dL

You should be able to check this on yourself right now. The bare minimum of health, in my opinion, is to get to these levels or slightly below. I will tell you the real numbers you want to achieve for optimal health in a group of important biomarkers.

If you remain insulin resistant, inflamed, and have high levels of AGEs and oxidative stress, you will have aches and pains, joint problems, stiffness, arthritis, tendinitis, fatigue, weakness, and just will not feel good at all. But all of this can be improved naturally, as you have learned.

WHAT'S MY INFLAMMATORY LOAD?

HsCRP stands for high-sensitivity c-reactive protein (CRP)—a protein made by your liver. Serum testing of hsCRP levels can give insight into your over-all inflammatory burden. You want a hsCRP because the regular CRP is just not good enough. It took years, but finally, the AHA and other societies have recognized that inflammation is a serious problem, and now the hsCRP is becoming more common.

What is considered to be normal in our population is <2 mg/L.
Optimal would be <1 mg/L, or really <0.5 mg/L.

WHAT DOES MY LIPID PANEL SHOW? (HDL, LDL, TRIGLYCERIDES)

The lipid panel monitors and screens for your risk of cardiovascular disease. Lipids also give insight into insulin resistance. This complete cholesterol test measures the amount of cholesterol and triglycerides in your blood. Standard teaching tells you that HDL (high-density lipoprotein) cholesterol is the good kind; LDL (low-density lipoprotein) is the bad kind. Triglycerides represent the most common type of fat in your body. VLDLs are very-low-density lipoproteins, and these are the carrier molecules for fat around the body. If they are unable to deliver their load to a cell because the cell is energy overloaded and insulin resistant, levels will build up in serum.

Fat stored inside a cell is the start of insulin resistance. Insulin resistance is now thought to begin in muscle, then liver, then to move on to diabetes. Fatty liver is a great sign that you have insulin resistance and are likely to get diabetes. If you have fatty liver or insulin resistance, as about 50 percent of Americans do, you will also have whole joint inflammatory disease. It is so important to get your diet right and to exercise to prevent or reverse insulin resistance if you want to have less pain.

What values do your regular doctors want to see on your report? In other words, what is normal for the American population?

Total cholesterol should be under 200.
HDL cholesterol should be over 60 (and the higher the better).
LDL cholesterol should be under 100 (and the lower the better).
Triglycerides should be under 150.

Lipids are extremely complex, and there are entire subspecialties of medicine devoted to this. I am just going to tell you what I would have you shoot for if you were my patient and reported achy joints, stiffness, overweight, fatigue, and the like to me.

Optimal cholesterol will be 100–199.
Optimal triglycerides should be 0–149; realistically, ≤100 is a good
    number to achieve.
HDL should be >39 or 40.
VLDL should be 5–40.
LDL should be 0–99.

To get even more detailed, look at your ApoB levels. These are proteins that attach to the VLDL and LDL particles for fatty transport.

A good number here would be ApoB = <90 mg.
Optimal is ApoB = <50 mg.

Insulin resistance is at the heart of many of our problems. Combined with chronic low-grade inflammation, glycation, and oxidative stress, it leads to all of your health problems. This means you have the power to fix a lot of what is wrong. One of the best things to understand is your personal glucose management.

A fasting glucose is what is normally checked. But understand that your pancreas (if you do not have type 1 diabetes mellitus) is pumping out massive amounts of insulin to make up for insulin resistance, and the glucose levels will not look terrible for years and years. But the problem has already started.

What is considered "normal" for fasting glucose? Your doctor will tell you that 100mg/L is okay. However, more and more research is proving that this level means you already have insulin resistance.

Ideal glucose is <90 mg/L.
Optimal is <80 mg/L.

If you can check your glucose levels after a meal (30–45 minutes later), it should not spike more than 115 mg/L in theory. The American Diabetes Association states that glucose should be ≤140 an hour or two after a meal.

WHAT'S MY A1C TEST SAY? (GLYCATED HEMOGLOBIN)

When sugar enters your bloodstream, it attaches to hemoglobin (a protein in your red blood cells) via the glycation reaction. Although everyone has some sugar attached to their hemoglobin, people with high blood sugar have more attached. This blood test (also known as the HbA1c test) is commonly used to diagnose, monitor, or control prediabetes and diabetes. The HbA1C level gives you the average of the three prior months' daily glucose levels.

Ideally, you would have a level < 5.0 percent

WHAT'S MY FASTING INSULIN LEVEL?

Prediabetes, diabetes, metabolic syndrome, and hypoglycemia are all serious conditions that can have a severe impact on how you live your daily life. Many people who have these conditions don't realize it because they develop over a long time. Diabetes, for example, starts with insulin resistance.

A fasting insulin level can show if your pancreas is putting out more insulin than it really should in an effort to make up for over-feeding and hyperglycemia. The purpose of the fasting insulin test (*not* the same as the fasting glucose test) is to detect signals trending toward pre-diabetes. The blood glucose and A1C tests prove very valuable, but the fasting insulin test picks up a problem much earlier. So this test is ideal to predict early signs of blood sugar problems. It is possible to do an insulin challenge test similar to the glucose challenge. This gives even more information.

Your fasting insulin is normal between 2 and 6 IU/mL; for optimal health it should really be < 3.

Another parameter that should be assessed is your HOMA-IR score. This is the homeostatic model assessment—insulin resistance. This is a good way to evaluate the relationship between your insulin and glucose levels. This is calculated as follows:

First, to convert from pmol/L to uIU/mL, divide by 6.
To convert from mmol/L to mg/dL, multiply by 18.
(Fasting insulin in uIU/mL × fasting glucose in mmol/L) / 22.5.
Alternatively, the formula can be (fasting insulin iuU/mL × fasting glucose mg/dL) / 405.

The answers should work out to be the same.

Less than 1.0 means you are insulin sensitive: this is good.

A number above 1.9 means you have early insulin resistance.

A number above 2.9 means you have insulin resistance.

WHAT'S MY URIC ACID LEVEL?

Uric acid is created when the body breaks down chemicals called purines. It is also formed when fructose is metabolized. Diets high in purines or fructose increase the level of uric acid: salmon, shrimp, lobster, red meat, organ meats like liver, and food with high-fructose corn syrup and alcoholic drinks (especially beer). Fructose is one of the primary drivers of uric acid in today's America. Most uric acid dissolves in the bloodstream, passes through the kidneys, and exits the body in urine.

Occasionally, however, it does not. Researchers have found a link between uric acid and type 2 diabetes, high blood pressure, and fatty liver disease. High uric acid can also cause crystals of uric acid to form, leading to kidney stones or gout (a painful form of arthritis). Gout is more and more commonly seen in the clinical setting.

A standard, normal uric acid is thought to be between 3.5 and
    7.0 mg/dL.

For optimal health, you should try to get your uric acid below 5.5
    and maybe even 5.9 mg/dL.

WHAT DOES MY ROUTINE BLOOD PRESSURE READING REVEAL?

Your blood pressure represents the force your heart uses to pump blood through the arteries as it travels through your body. The optimal level varies by age, but the ideal for adults ranges between 90/60 and 120/80. "High" blood pressure is considered to be 140/90 or higher. "Low" blood pressure is considered to be lower than 90/60.

The top number is the systolic pressure. The lower number is the diastolic pressure. Both are important, but they measure different things. The top number measures the pressure in your arteries when your heart beats. The bottom number measures the pressure in your arteries when your heart rests between beats. Most studies show a greater risk of stroke and heart disease is related to the higher systolic (top) number as compared to the elevated diastolic (bottom) number.

The higher your blood pressure, the more risk you have for heart disease, heart attack, or stroke. A heart attack, heart failure, heart valve disease, and an extremely low heart rate (bradycardia) can cause low blood pressure.

If you're healthy with low blood pressure and have no symptoms, that's typically not something to worry about. You don't need treatment. But low blood pressure can be a sign of an underlying problem like inadequate blood flow to the heart, brain, or other vital organs. So definitely, if you start to have symptoms (dizziness, nausea, dehydration, blurred vision, weakness, confusion, fainting, cold/clammy pale skin), you should have your doctor investigate the cause.

When your blood pressure consistently ranges 140/90 or higher, you will definitely need to make lifestyle changes (diet, exercise, sleep, stress relief)—or take medications to lower the pressure. High blood pressure is also associated with arthritis and painful joints as well.

Normal is systolic <120 mmHg, diastolic <80 mmHg.

Borderline is systolic 120–129, diastolic <80.

Hypertension stage 1 is systolic 130–139 mmHg, diastolic 80–89 mmHg.

Hypertension stage 2 is systolic 140 mmHg, diastolic >90 mmHg.

Hypertension stage 3 is systolic >180 mmHg, diastolic >120 mmHg.

WHAT DOES THE DEXA TEST TELL ME ABOUT BONE DENSITY?

If you have osteoporosis, you may not know it until you break a brittle bone. There are no other symptoms to create awareness. However, a doctor may notice this condition when taking an X-ray for other reasons.

You should be tested periodically to measure your bone mineral density and take preventative steps. The DEXA (dual-energy X-ray absorptiometry) scan lets you know the state of your bones. Although there's no cure for osteoporosis, you can slow the bone-thinning process and rebuild new bone with resistance exercise. There are some newer biologic drugs that do add bone over time, but normally, only older bisphosphonates are covered by insurance companies.

Remember, bone can heal itself, and new growth of bone cells strengthen the bone. But this process to grow new bone takes months. So it's far better to become aware of deteriorating bone and prevent further loss and osteoporosis. Fun fact: bone is one of few tissues that heals without scar. The first steps toward strong bones: exercise, keeping your blood pressure at optimal levels, stopping smoking, and getting more calcium, magnesium, D3, and K2 through your foods or supplements.

The DEXA scan is scored based on your bone density compared to normal thirty-year-olds. You will receive a T-score and be graded on that. These studies are covered by most insurance companies every three years or so.

Normal is between +1 and –1.

If your T-score is between –1 and –2.5 you have osteopenia, but not osteoporosis yet.

If your score is –2.5 or lower, you have osteoporosis.

I am sad to say that I have seen many patients with a T-score of –2.5 who are not medicated for osteoporosis, nor are they lifting weights. If you get a DEXA, make sure you have some follow-up care for the results.

WHAT'S MY CARDIAC CALCIUM SCORE?

As people age, they tend to develop calcified plaque in their heart and arteries. Your score on this test reflects the amount of calcification in coronary arteries, which might indicate arterial inflammation. There are even more sensitive tests for that, but you can get a CT for cardiac calcium score pretty easily in most communities. You just need to ask your doctor to order it. A score of zero means no calcium is present. That's the ideal and normal score. That low score suggests a low chance of developing a heart attack.

If the test shows calcium deposits, the higher the score, the higher your risk for heart disease. The calcium scores have the highest validity if you have not already had a heart attack or received a stent. Another thing to keep in mind: These scores are only reliable for men forty and over and women over the age of fifty. Some people who exercise intensely have calcium buildup in arteries that is actually protective.

If your cardiac calcium score is high, a proper diet and exercise can help. If those don't lower the score, you may need medications or procedures to remove the plaque buildup.

I often order these studies for my patients. I am prompted to do so by the many people I see for lower back pain that have a calcified aorta on their spine films. The aorta is the great vessel that leaves the heart and brings blood to the periphery. My assumption is that if it calcified, the coronary arteries must be as well. This is also a mark for peripheral arterial disease.

A score of zero means that you have a low chance of a future heart attack.

A score of 100–300 indicates higher risk of heart disease.

A score of ≥300 is a sign of very high risk of future heart disease.

DO I HAVE ANY TOXIC METALS IN MY SYSTEM?

In my experience practicing Western medicine, the concept of heavy-metal toxicity is not taken very seriously.

Toxic metals tend to distribute widely through the body. The general complaints of fatigue and weakness are due to the damage on mitochondria and cell membranes from, you guessed it, oxidative stress caused by the metals.

The most common heavy metals in humans are mercury, lead, or cadmium. Typically, you might get exposed to high concentrations of these metals from food or food containers with defective coating, air or water pollution, lead-based paint, industrial exposure, or even medicine. Although the regulators and government have told you there are "safe" levels of these heavy metals, most of them should really be at zero as there is no physiologic reason for them to be in the system at all.

Your doctor can check for heavy metal poisoning with a simple blood test known as a heavy metals panel or a heavy metal toxicity test. This is really all that is available to you without paying cash for specialized lab tests.

If you have symptoms of heavy metal poisoning (diarrhea, nausea, abdominal pain, vomiting, shortness of breath, tingling in your hands or feet, chills, weakness) but your blood test shows only low metal levels, you might need additional testing to identify a problem:

- Liver function studies
- Kidney function tests
- Urine analysis
- Fingernail analysis
- Hair analysis
- Electrocardiogram
- X-rays

Do keep in mind that the above symptoms are common symptoms for many conditions and causes. So this basic testing will be the quickest, most direct way to know if your symptoms are due to toxic metals. I often order a heavy-metal profile for my patients. There are more accurate ways to measure, but this is all that insurance will cover and is easy for patients to do. The levels that are considered normal are as follows:

- Lead: 0.0–3.4 ug/dL
- Arsenic: 0–9 ug/L
- Mercury: 0.0–14.9 ug/L
- Cadmium: 0.0–1.2 ug/L
- Manganese: 0.0–18.3 ug/L
- Copper: 70–155 ug/dL
- Zinc: 60.0–120.0 ug/dL
- Selenium: 23.0–190.0 ug/L
- Cobalt: 0.0–1.8 ug/L
- Chromium: 0.0–5.0 ng/L

Even these "normal" levels vary by laboratory, and sometimes by gender and age. Check your local laboratory's actual reference range if you plan on testing.

For mild toxicity, you might be able to solve the problem by eliminating your exposure to heavy metal or by altering your diet. I often tell my patients not to eat oysters more than once a month, nor sushi for this reason.

It is thought that regular consumption of certain herbs can diminish the absorption of toxic metals. Fiber, such as pectin, also reduces toxicity of these metals. Metals like to bind sulfurs, and thus, diets filled with garlic, onion, and the brassica vegetables will also provide protection. Another great and tasty herb that can reduce absorption of heavy metals is cilantro. Ginkgo and turmeric also have properties to protect from metal toxicity.

One of the best ways to remove heavy metals from your body is through sweating. The sauna is a very good way to do this. More heavy metals are excreted by the body through sweat than through urine or feces.

LIVER TESTS

Insulin resistance is a huge problem in our country. Remember: about 50 percent of us have this, but many remain asymptomatic with initially normal blood glucose. Your liver health is a peek into your overall health. If your liver is not working properly, your joints, muscle, bone, connective tissues, and other musculoskeletal tissues will not work well either. Fatty liver is a sign of insulin resistance. Fatty liver will alter your biomarkers in certain ways, even while you may be asymptomatic.

Here is what you should look for in your bloodwork: AST, ALT, and GGT.

Alanine aminotransferase (ALT) normal range is 7–55 iu/L.
Aspartate aminotransferase (AST) normal range is 8–48 iu/L.
Gamma-glutamyl transferase (GGT) normal range is 0–30 iu/L.

Normally, AST will be lower than ALT. As you can see, the ranges are quite large. The ratio of AST:ALT is often considered when looking at liver health. GGT is quite specific for liver injury and disease.

Optimal AST for men should be 14 to 20; for women it should be
    10–36.
Optimal ALT would be 9 to 14.

If you have acute liver injury, there will be a spike in the ALT. Chronic liver disease means that other organs are beginning to be affected and AST will go up as well. Most clinicians only consider a level to be elevated, however, if it is double or triple the "normal" amount.

A normal ratio of AST:ALT should be <1.

VITAMINS AND MICRONUTRIENTS

First, you should be aware that it is difficult to really get a good handle on your micronutrient and vitamin status. Most blood tests are inaccurate as many of these molecules are stored in tissues. However, I will give you some general guidelines here to help with your achy joints!

Most Americans, of course, are deficient in basic molecules of nutrition. Remember, ultraprocessed foods extract all of these during the processing. This is why you see breakfast cereal with words like "9 essential vitamins and minerals added." That is because they add these at the end in a vain attempt to make the cereal more foodlike.

About 94 percent of Americans are deficient in vitamin D3; 92 percent are deficient in choline; 67 percent are deficient in vitamin K; 56 to 60 percent are deficient in magnesium; 44 percent are deficient in calcium; 43 percent are deficient in vitamin A; and 89 percent are deficient in vitamin E.

Considering that our "normal" levels are set so low, this is quite frightening in my opinion.

So what levels should we have in our blood? Here is a short list:

- Optimal D3 should be 45–50 ng/ml, really closer to 70 or 80 ng/ml if you are an athlete.
- Optimal B12 should be around 180 pg/ml–914 pg/ml.
- Optimal magnesium should be 1.7 mg/dL–2.2 mg/dL.
- Optimal zinc should be 0.66 ug/ml–1.10 ug/ml.
- Optimal vitamin C should be 0.2–20. mg/dL.
- Optimal vitamin E should be 5 ug/dL–25 mg/dL.
- Optimal vitamin A should be 30 ug/dL–80 ug/dL.
- Optimal folic acid should be 2.6 ug/L–12.2 ug/L.
- Optimal selenium should be 23.0 ug/L–190.0 ug/L.
- Optimal copper should be 70–150 ug/dL.
- Optimal CoQ10 should be 0.4–1.6 mg/L.
- Vitamin B1 should be 90 nmol/L–140 nmol/L.

- Vitamin B6 should be 5 ng/ml–25 ng/ml.
- Vitamin K should be 0.13 ng/ml–1.19 ng/ml.

INSIST ON SHARED DECISION-MAKING

True shared decision-making means your doctor educates you about the details of your condition or decision; about the diagnosis and supporting reasoning; about the pros and cons of any recommended testing, surgeries, medicines, or other treatments. They should also discuss with you the statistics on the success rate of recommended testing, surgeries, medicines, and other treatments; other available options to deal with your condition (such as natural treatments, therapies, diets, supplements, exercises). You should ask how to ensure a smooth recovery. In an ideal world, you would discuss mindset and sleep as well.

Caring doctors have good intentions, but they may offer only a brief explanation to support their recommendations. They may think either you won't understand their explanations or you trust them explicitly to "do what's best." Truly, they probably just run out of time.

Trusting your doctor is good, even necessary. But doctors rarely have opportunity to know your complete profile and life situation.

Your doctor does not know your complete profile: your health goals, your life goals, your work requirements and conditions, your financial means, your endurance, your pain tolerance, your self-discipline, your patience or impatience, or your family situation and responsibilities. Unless they understand all these things, their recommendations will necessarily be limited.

If your doctor works for a hospital or for a large group they are likely forced to limit testing. One of the unspoken problems of the Affordable Care Act are the Accountable Care Organizations (ACOs) to which such doctors belong. In these operations, if a system saves money the hospital and doctors receive a bonus payment. This means that if they order fewer tests, they get a bonus. You really need to advocate for yourself. You have the bigger picture. Giving yourself agency in your own healthcare decisions improves your chances of success many times over.

With complete information from your doctor and your own research, you can feel competent and confident about making healthcare decisions *with* your doctor.

Chapter Ten

THE WARNER PROTOCOL
TO FEEL BETTER

As a doctor, I'm most concerned about preventing a serious condition or disease before it develops. So here's my protocol to revolutionize your health in a matter of months, not years. It's important that you know that it is okay if it takes a couple of years to fully incorporate the whole protocol into your life. Each step alone will provide immense benefits. It's the combination of the steps that give you the synergistic and exponential health results. I did not start this protocol until recently myself, and it took a while to get everything in place.

The protocol consists of a series of lifestyle changes to incorporate at your own pace. If your job, family, or other factors keep you from doing one of the steps, please don't give up. Simply engage the other aspects of the protocol, and you should still see dramatic benefits.

The steps don't have to be followed in exact order. However, I believe sleep is so foundational to human health that I emphasize that as the first step. That said, this is hard to get right, and I don't want you to be frustrated if you don't achieve a perfect, nonfragmented, nine-hour sleep experience each night. I personally haven't yet, but I'm not giving up and will continue with my protocol. Here are the steps:

- Good sleep
- Circadian rhythm
- Time-restricted eating
- Mediterranean diet pattern
- Exercise, especially resistance
- Mindset and stress control
- Supplements
- Adjunctive methods

Let's discuss these in a summarized fashion. This will help you to remember all that you have learned, so you can incorporate it into your life.

SLEEP

- Get a sleep study. This is one of the first things I order for patients seeking to feel less pain and improve their overall health. Most have issues with sleep, and this information is very helpful. If your physician won't order one, find another!
- Get a minimum of seven to nine hours of quality sleep each night. This is not negotiable. There are few people, if any, who don't require the full amount of time for the brain to drain toxins via the glymphatic system and for the body to do all the repair and restoration needed to function and feel good the next day. All memories and other aspects of neuroplasticity tend to happen during sleep as well.
- Remember that light is the suppression signal for melatonin. Begin dimming lights in the house around 5:00 or 6:00 p.m. Then bright lights, or sunlight, when you wake up trigger cortisol.
- Cool rooms are healthy for sleep and the stress-response system. Optimal sleep temperature is around 65 Fahrenheit.
- Try to limit all stimulants after 12:00 p.m. Remember: caffeine has a half-life of twelve hours.

- Sleep hinges on a good circadian rhythm, so that can be worked on at the same time.

CIRCADIAN RHYTHM

This might be one of the most life-changing parts of my protocol.

- Establish a set bedtime that works for you, your family, and your work. Early bedtimes are best. For example, try to be in bed and going to sleep around 9:00 p.m. Then try to wake up at a time that correlates to the bedtime, such as 5:00 or 6:00 a.m. This provides eight or nine hours of sleep. The key is to maintain the same daily schedule, within a half-hour or so, on a regular basis. There should not be a variance on the weekends—that can introduce social jet lag.
- Do not deviate. The routine and stringency will reduce your stress over time. Routine works well for the human condition.

By establishing a solid routine, you'll find over time that every system in your body feels better. You will develop a good cortisol-melatonin balance and relationship. You will allow the myriad clock genes in your muscle, bone, joints, ligaments, and so on to function correctly and at the times they should to optimize your body.

Likewise, your joints will be able to repair damage and restore tissue to your benefit. Your mood and stress and resiliency will also be optimized. There will be far less pain by simply allowing a rhythm to life.

TIME-RESTRICTED EATING

TRE is a necessary corollary to your circadian rhythm. Remember: there are signals from the suprachiasmatic nucleus (the brain's master clock) with light exposure to promote levels of cortisol and also melatonin (when there is an absence of light). Cortisol is a messenger to the body that the day has started. Melatonin tells the body to rest, repair, restore, and sleep. The light-based signaling to the peripheral clock genes must be accompanied by the same gut-derived signals. There is a feeding-based clock in the gut that signals to your peripheral tissues. This clock must match the master clock of the brain. Therefore, you must eat within a certain window of time that matches your circadian rhythm.

It's best to wait at least an hour after waking to eat and not to eat within a few hours of sleeping. Obviously, not everyone will achieve a "perfect" schedule. Good news: no one knows what the perfect schedule is. Based on my experience and interpretation of all the studies I have read over the years, and my understanding of the practicalities of most lives, a twelve-to-twelve or fourteen-to-ten (fasting to eating) schedule is fine. I don't think we all have to do sixteen-hour fasts and only eat during an eight-hour window. I also believe that daily time-restricted eating makes more sense over a life than intermittent fasting. I imagine that not eating for a full day or two would really change the gut-derived clock signals to your tissues. The fast that you allow your body prompts all of the detoxification, healing, and repair to happen. If the body senses nutrients, it will not go into the stress-response and repair mode.

The easiest way to start this lifestyle practice is the twelve-to-twelve schedule. I tell my patients who are interested to only eat/drink between 8:00 a.m. and 8:00 p.m. to start (for example). Once this becomes routine and easy, they can lop off an hour or two and hit the fourteen-hour fast and ten-hour feeding schedule.

There are a lot of nuances as to what "breaks a fast" and such. I'm not going to open that can of worms here. Just try to match a reasonable window of eating with a good fasting window and your circadian rhythm. I personally believe about 50 percent of joint pain goes away just doing this.

TRE, even with a crappy diet, can change a lot of your health parameters for the better. This is a very important part of the protocol. If you can sleep well, establish a good circadian rhythm, and a solid TRE schedule, then incorporate a good dietary pattern, I predict you'll wonder why you ever did anything differently.

MEDITERRANEAN DIET PATTERN

It bears repeating that the body of evidence for this lifestyle and eating pattern is substantial and points to how it treats most NCDs, including arthritis. Most people with this lifestyle have less pain, better function, and fewer chronic diseases than others and live longer and are happier. There are a million diets out there, and each has its merits. But for overall approachability, effectiveness, and sustainability, in my opinion there is no better pattern to follow.

- Avoid ultraprocessed foods whenever possible. I understand this is difficult in America, but even avoiding it sometimes puts you in a new health category. Always avoid fast food—it has no redeeming health or nutritional qualities.

- Try to consume extra-virgin olive oil as much as possible. This monounsaturated fat is anti-inflammatory and antioxidant and provides myriad health benefits. Try to replace seed and vegetable oils with olive oil when you can.

- Make sure you eat as many vegetables and whole fruits (no juices!) along with whole grains. Not all carbs are bad. In fact, most of them are great if they aren't overly processed, and include some fiber. The relative amount of fiber is important in combination with carbohydrates.

- Consume very little, if any, added sugar or fructose. Just avoiding added sugars provides a lot of the anti-inflammatory and glucose-regulating benefits of any diet.

- Limit alcohol intake. It's metabolized along the same pathway as fructose and is just empty calories. That said, alcohol has been part of human society for thousands of years and will continue as such. Just be mindful.

- Pay attention to how you cook your meals. Be thoughtful and present as you cook. Ideally, cook with friends and family whenever possible. Social connection is one of the reasons this lifestyle is so effective.

- Use spices and herbs to flavor your food liberally. Each and every culinary herb has a health benefit.

- Make sure to eat plenty of wild-caught seafood or supplement with omega-3 fatty acids. The omega-3 fatty acids definitely reduce inflammation in the body and brain. They also increase flexibility and the basic functionality of all cells.
- Supplement your diet if you know it doesn't provide you with an ample supply of necessary nutrients to prevent common conditions or reverse painful or harmful conditions and diseases. Supplementation with specific nutrients can help orthopedic conditions.

EXERCISE

The importance of exercise for the health of the mind and body can't be overstated. To date, no drug has beat the outcomes of exercise for almost all conditions. It improves not just the function of your body, but also your brain. Movement is key to longevity and a properly working body, pain reduction, and the treatment of arthritis, and other musculoskeletal problems.

All reputable clinical guidelines recommend exercise as a first-line treatment for arthritis.

- Start small if you must, and build strength and endurance as you can. There is not one single program or type of exercise that is better than any other to improve the signs and symptoms of arthritis and other orthopedic problems. It is more important that you start moving in any way that you can. Eventually, you'll progress and do more. For example, if you just get up from the desk five minutes every hour and walk around the office, you have added forty minutes of movement to the day. Perhaps eventually, you'll be running up the stairs at the office for twenty-second bursts twice a day (shown to be very beneficial for health).
- Seek guidance if you need help. A competent physical therapist, physician, or trainer can assess your medical conditions, limitations, beliefs, and attitudes about exercise, and any contraindications to a particular activity and design a program for you to follow. I have personally

helped wheelchair-bound eighty-five-year-olds develop the strength and skills to do curls, take walks, and need less assistance for daily activities. All of this is possible because the body never loses the ability to add muscle strength and endurance. It just takes some effort.

- Exercise consistently for 120–150 minutes each week performed at the zone 2 level. That is, you should be exerting yourself but still able to have a conversation, albeit one of few words. This is about thirty minutes daily for five days and can be broken into three ten-minute blocks as we stated before. There are no hard-and-fast rules. Just begin moving. Any movement is better than no movement, do not get hung up on the numbers.

- Plan to do both cardio exercises (walking, biking, swimming, and so forth) as well as resistance and strength training (weights). Try to do this with a friend or a group if you like. This will increase the social connectivity and relationship building that is vital for longevity.

- Resistance work is crucial for a body to feel great and for longevity. Strength improvement can be made with a simple protocol. Just doing three to five movements with load for three to five repetitions just three to five days a week can build strength. The movements need to involve resisting a load that is about 70–80 percent of your one-repetition maximum ability. Or get an appointment with a physical therapist for help. This recipe for strength may only take twenty minutes three times each week.

- Choose an exercise you enjoy and that your schedule and family will accommodate. Your activity does not have to involve expensive equipment, streaming memberships, gym memberships, or anything else. Simple body-weight resistance and walking is enough to benefit your body and make you feel better.

- Don't be scared of protein. Sarcopenia is a scourge and should be avoided. Eat enough protein to maintain your body and then add some to build more muscle. The general guidelines are about 0.35 g of protein per pound of body weight for maintenance. A two-hundred-pound person should eat 70 g of protein daily. This goes up if you do some resistance work. A lot of the pain and dysfunction found in an orthopedic clinic waiting room could be treated with just the addition of some muscle.

MINDSET

There is an enormous amount of money being spent on government contracts and corporate consulting deals to teach people to have optimistic mindsets, to be resilient, and to change catastrophic and negative thinking. I've found over years of life that if you follow the money, you find the truth. Mindset work is a fundamental right to all people, not just Fortune 500 CEOs and tech billionaires. You can pursue such a practice on your own with a few simple tricks. Obviously, you can always seek a referral to a competent psychologist to assist in this endeavor. I really just want you to understand how important mindset is to how your body feels, brain works, and to your longevity and happiness. After all, the pursuit of happiness is a goal, right?

- Forget everything you know about how healthcare matters are "supposed to work." You're not "supposed to" have hip replacements, knee replacements, back pain, or muscle aches just because you're living longer. The fact that you even have such thoughts is proof that you've been tricked into what is called learned helplessness. You've been taught to lack agency when it comes to how your body feels and how your joints and muscles work. Get rid of these thoughts. I have taught you about sham surgeries, asymptomatic MRI findings, and the geographic nature of most treatment decisions. You should realize by now that most of what you're told is probably smoke and mirrors.

- To emphasize, forget what your MRI shows. Review chapter 1 about abnormalities showing up in scans for people with no symptoms, as well as those with symptoms. Forget about the indisputable effectiveness of surgery and drugs. Check statistics about positive outcomes of various invasive procedures and strong pharmaceuticals before proceeding.

- Investigate the preferences for certain surgeries based on your geographic locale. You may discover your surgery has been recommended not because of your symptoms but because of referral networks that provide financial incentives, or even simply because of groupthink.

- Get a second or third opinion before agreeing to complex, expensive treatments, procedures, and surgeries. Most surgical decisions are based on habit, groupthink, or similar organizational behavior problems. Knowing this is a good thing. Keep it in mind.

- Take charge of your healthcare and healthcare education. Do not let your healthcare providers treat you like a child when it comes to facts, information, and reasoning. Also understand that an AI program will be making most of your healthcare decisions going forward, especially as it pertains to coverage for care by your insurance company. The problem with AI—one of many—is that bad data in means bad data out. Be very aware of how pervasive this technology is becoming in the back offices of your insurance company.

- Stop thinking catastrophically about your pain, stiffness, swelling, or weakness! Don't think an injury is the end of the world. This is hugely important. You have learned how pain catastrophizing directly controls symptoms, outcomes, and the overall orthopedic condition. Become self-aware and recognize when negative thoughts and emotions are out of proportion to your medical condition.

- Learn to think optimistically. The biggest difference between resilient people and those that have learned helplessness is the level of optimism. And, yes, you can train yourself to think more positively about everything. How people react to injury, pain, impairment, and the like is distributed on a bell curve much like all else in life. Those at the left side of the curve give up and give in (learned helplessness), while those in the middle—the majority of us—will have some depression for a while but will eventually get back in the game and work on things. Those at the far-right side of the curve are the true optimists and super-resilient. Like the middle and largest group of people, they may have temporary depression and listlessness with a problem, but then they take it as an opportunity to become even better than before. I want you at least in the middle group and, hopefully beginning to be on the right side of the curve.

- Find and participate in a supportive group to minimize stress, enjoy social relationships, and improve your mental health. Loneliness is one of our great and silent killers, and also increases pain and other symptoms of arthritis. Find something bigger than yourself to engage in and get your spiritual side growing. This doesn't have to be religion; just find something that has actual meaning and gives purpose. This can range from reading a book to a child to volunteering for Habitat for Humanity. Think about something that matters to you and get involved. Mindset masters know that it is mandatory to have a wide perspective on life and to avoid self-absorption. True happiness and flow come when we are completely focused on a larger purpose.

- Believe in yourself and your actions. This is agency. Know in your heart that if you start living a healthier lifestyle, you'll definitely feel better. There is no evidence that healthy lifestyles are bad for you anywhere in anything I have seen, heard, or read. There is a reason that healthy people tend to look younger, act younger, perform well, have less pain, and are generally not obese. Granted, as I said, only about 10 percent of our country is metabolically healthy, but I want you in that group.

This protocol is meant to be a guide. Add each step as you're able. If you don't achieve perfection at each step, don't worry. You'll be doing your brain and body a world of favors even instituting just a *part* of *one* of the steps. If you can do all of the steps and then make that your lifestyle, I predict a happy, healthy you with a long life full of grace. Each portion of this protocol is synergistic with the others. Take a stepwise approach and enjoy it. Incorporating my Well Theory Protocol into your life is not meant to cause mental stress! Rather, each step of the MEDS can be taken in part and slowly. I understand how hard it is to change a routine and lifestyle in modern America. If you get the mindset right, the TRE and better diet will be easier to start. If you get a better diet, the mindset will be easier to harness. If you begin to exercise, the mindset will also come easier. Meanwhile, a healthy mindset makes exercise more enjoyable. Sleep allows for all of your tissues and your brain to rest, repair, and restore themselves. Better sleep makes a better mindset and makes exercise easier. Better sleep, respecting a circadian rhythm, reduces stress and improves resiliency. A better diet allows for all the micronutrients and antioxidants that provide tools for the body to repair itself as you sleep. I could go on and on about the interplay and benefits of each aspect of MEDS, but I think you get it by now!

So there you have it: My protocol to transform your health, avoid surgery, fight aging, reduce stress, lose weight, lower inflammation, and live well. It's your life—make it count!

—Dr. Meredith Warner

APPENDIX I

LIST OF SUPPLEMENTS

DISCLAIMER: I DO NOT RECOMMEND ANY OF THE FOLLOWING SUPPLEMENTS FOR PREGNANT WOMEN, BREASTFEEDING WOMEN, OR CHILDREN. PLEASE CONSULT YOUR PHYSICIAN BEFORE TAKING ANY SUPPLEMENTS.

Alpha-Lipoic Acid

Benefits

- Breaks down carbohydrates (glucose metabolism) to create energy and help control symptoms of type 2 diabetes
- Curbs appetite, helping with weight control and pain management
- Fights chronic inflammation by increasing your antioxidant intake and cellular health
- Helps protect the brain
- Helps with certain liver diseases
- Helps to counteract alcohol metabolism

- Specific antioxidant for neural tissues
- As a lipophilic and hydrophilic antioxidant, ALA is highly protective of nerve and connective-tissue function. It will help to control pain, especially nerve-based pain.

Foods: Red meat, carrots, beets, spinach, broccoli, potatoes, yams, yeast, tomatoes, brussels sprouts, rice bran

Daily Dosage: 600–1,800 mg

Warnings: Side effects are typically rare, but could include insomnia, fatigue, diarrhea, or skin rash. Because it can lower blood sugar, diabetics should take this only after talking with their doctor.

Basil

Benefits
- Aids digestion
- Fights inflammation and free radical activity
- Helps with depression
- Aids in managing diabetes by lowering glucose
- Decreases levels of cortisol and helps with stress management
- Helps to reduce pain through the actions of eugenol, a phytochemical in basil and cloves
- Supports liver function and helps to detoxify your body
- Cleanses the kidneys and lowers uric acid
- Is high in vitamin K, which reduces the risk of atherosclerosis and also supports bone health, along with vitamin D3, calcium, and magnesium.

Daily Dosage: 300–2,000 mg (the usual recommendation is 500 mg daily)

Warnings: Side effects include slow blood clotting and increased risk of bleeding disorders. It has caused cancer in mice. Basil can interfere with blood-thinning drugs.

Bay Leaf

Benefits

- Shown to reduce tumor growth in some cancers
- Highly antioxidant; more powerful than synthetic antioxidants or vitamin C
- Traditional remedy for symptoms of osteoarthritis
- Acts as an anti-inflammatory to reduce pain from musculoskeletal conditions

Black Pepper

Benefits

- Increases the bioavailability of turmeric through the substance piperine
- Treats arthritis by reducing levels of damaging proinflammatory molecules
- Preclinical studies demonstrated an ability to enhance cognition and reduce depression

Berberine

Benefits

- May help strengthen your heart health by effects on lipids
- Decreases insulin resistance

- Regulates how the body uses sugar; considered as powerful as metformin in this regard
- Assists with metabolic health in conditions such as diabetes and obesity; in turn this helps with the associated problems of arthritis, tendinitis, and pain
- Helps regulate serum lipid levels
- Fights several bacterial infections, including sepsis, pneumonia, meningitis, and several skin conditions
- Reduces swelling
- Will help to reduce the amount of AGEs that are deposited in your body

Foods: None

Daily Dosage: 1,000–1,500 mg

Warnings/Deficiency/Overdose/Side Effects: Side effects include diarrhea, constipation, gas, and stomach pain. Because it can reduce blood sugar, in high doses, it may increase the risk for hypoglycemia.

Bromelain[1]

Benefits
- This is a strong anti-inflammatory from the pineapple plant. It decreases levels of certain painful prostaglandins. It is also a source of protease inhibitors and prevents cartilage breakdown.
- Reduces pain from arthritis
- Fibrinolytic, slows clotting
- Can relax muscles and provide comfort from muscle pain

Daily Dosage: 45–1,200 mg daily; there is no consensus and doses as high as 2,000 mg daily have been used.

CBD (without THC, the Psychoactive Agent)

Benefits

- May help lower inflammation, by interacting with the endocannabinoid system to block pain receptors and calm the sensation of pain
- May help reduce neuropathic pain (common with diabetes, prediabetes, multiple sclerosis, herniated discs, and chemotherapy). Such pain is caused by damaged or dysfunctional nerves. CBD is up to twenty times more potent than NSAIDs, which can damage the heart and cause digestive upset.
- May aid in sleep by decreasing the release of cortisol, a critical hormone in the sleep-wake cycle. Higher cortisol levels mean alertness. Lower levels help you go to sleep faster and feel more rested upon waking.
- Regulates mood to reduce stress and anxiety by decreasing cortisol and by increasing serotonin
- Provides terpenes, which are a group of chemical compounds found in the hemp plant (conveys the unique smell of the plant) that can have anticancer, antimicrobial, antifungal, and anti-inflammatory benefits. A combination of terpenes with a dose of cannabinoids can create a noticeable enhancement of its therapeutic effect, often called the "entourage effect."

Daily Needs or Dosage: 25–100 mg routinely with little or no negative effect. Prescription level ranging from 500–800 mg (controls seizure disorders).

Warnings: Make sure any CBD product is tested for purity by a third-party and is produced inside the United States.

Celery Seed

Benefits

- Provides apigenin and other phytochemicals that help reduce inflammation
- Reduces activity of cyclooxygenase enzymes and, thus, inflammation
- Can reduce the frequency and severity of gout attacks
- Also known to reduce menstrual cramp pain, decrease LDL levels, decrease triglyceride levels, and protect the liver from toxicity
- Known as a natural diuretic

Chili Peppers (Capsaicin)

Benefits

- Pain relief: through heat and pain receptors, chili peppers can reduce symptoms of nerve pain along with pain from arthritis. Capsaicin is the active ingredient. Topical applications are the most recommended.
- Proven to help reduce chronic pain from neuropathy, radiculopathy, and nerve sources[2]
- Capsaicin will also reduce appetite, reduce postprandial glucose levels and can increase metabolism.
- Topical applications are also helpful to reduce symptoms of psoriasis

Chondroitin

Benefits

- Reduces joint pain and the swelling accompanying osteoarthritis by decreasing inflammation
- Aids in the regeneration of cartilage in knees and hip joints and repairs damaged cartilage; it is known to reduce joint deterioration

- A glycosaminoglycan, one of the main elements of the musculoskel-etal system. Chondroitin sulfate simply has an added sulfate group.

Daily Dosage: 800–1,500 mg

Warnings: Common side effects include nausea, diarrhea or constipation, heartburn, and intestinal gas. This supplement may interfere with the antico-agulant drug warfarin.

Cinnamon

Benefits
- Improves insulin function. Lowers blood glucose levels; Cinnamal-dehyde is an active ingredient shown to lower HbA1C (AGE) levels.
- Cinnamon is also highly antioxidant; it reduces that activity of the COX enzymes
- Helps control symptoms of irritable bowel syndrome or other diges-tive problems
- Works as an insect repellent (in topical ointment form); it is antibac-terial and antiviral
- Other active constituents are eugenol, linalool, and camphor

Daily Dosage: 1–2 tsp/day (2–6 g per day)

Warnings: An overdose can cause digestive problems or allergic reactions. Cassia cinnamon may contain small amounts of coumarin. Ceylon cinnamon has much less of this.

Clove

Benefits
- Clove is extremely antibacterial, antiviral, and antimicrobial. It is used in dental creams, toothpastes, mouthwashes, and wound salves.
- Eugenol is the active ingredient and is able to reduce pain associated with osteoarthritis, tendinitis, and other orthopedic problems
- Clove is very analgesic, antioxidant, numbing, and anti-inflammatory
- Clove and clove oil have been successful in treating joint and muscle pain, muscle spasm, indigestion and nausea, bloating; also, a strong agent to prevent infections.

CoQ10 (Coenzyme Q10)

Benefits
- Aids in treating symptoms of heart disease, diabetes, migraines, Parkinson's, periodontal disease, high blood pressure, myalgia, and statin-induced muscle pain
- Essential for the health of all tissues and organs; required for proper mitochondrial function. It is an electron shuttle for energy production.
- Reduces signs of aging by preventing damage caused by free radicals and oxidative stress
- Generates and helps recycle other antioxidants like vitamin E
- Reduces migraine symptoms
- Affects lipid composition and supports optimal functional of the cardiovascular system, the immune system, and the nervous system
- Impedes diabetic complications
- Reduces muscle pain caused by statin medications

Foods: Organ meats (heart, liver, kidney), pork, beef, chicken, fatty fish (trout, herring, salmon, mackerel, sardines), spinach, cauliflower, broccoli, oranges, strawberries, soybeans, lentils, peanuts, sesame seeds, pistachios

Daily Dosage: 150–200 mg

Warnings: Deficiencies damage and even destroy muscle cells. Although CoQ10 is typically found throughout the body in the heart, liver, kidneys, spleen, pancreas, and adrenal glands, deficiencies may develop because of nutritional problems, genetic defects, illness, and aging—all of which can significantly decrease CoQ10 levels. The most common cause of a deficiency is statin medication.

Fiber

Benefits[3]
- Lowers risk of dying from cardiac disease, stroke, type 2 diabetes, and colon cancer
- May lower cholesterol
- Improves glycemic control
- Normalizes stools in irritable bowel syndrome, preventing diarrhea and constipation
- Helps to normalize and maintain weight loss
- Supports a healthy gut biome
- Dietary fiber is either soluble or insoluble; both are needed.

Foods: Whole grains and cereals, whole fruits, whole vegetables

Daily Needs or Dosage: 25–38 g (most Americans eat only about 15 g a day)

Warnings: Fiber can cause gastrointestinal symptoms like bloating. Be sure to drink enough water when consuming fiber.

The best way to supplement is with psyllium husk, as this provides both soluble and insoluble fiber. Both are needed for proper gut health. With a good gut, the gut biome will produce the molecules needed to reduce the aches and pains of your orthopedic conditions.

GABA (Gamma-Aminobutyric Acid)

Benefits

- Aids the normal work of the nervous system; reduces the activity of the excitatory neurotransmitter glutamate. This reduces pain and hypersensitivity. Mediates presynaptic inhibition of sensory fibers.
- Calms the brain due to the lower activity from neurons, reducing stress and promoting relaxation; GABA is an inhibitory amino acid neurotransmitter.
- Aids sleep; receptors are found in the brain's sleep regulation area
- Enhances the immune system. Increases levels of growth hormone and insulin
- Pain from neuropathy is reduced by taking GABA.

Foods: Teas (green, black, oolong), tomatoes, chestnuts, mushrooms, spinach, broccoli, cabbage, cauliflower, brussels sprouts, sweet potatoes, fermented food products

Daily Dosage: 100–1,000 mg

Warnings: Side effects of GABA include upset stomach, headache, sleepiness, and muscle weakness.

Ginger

Benefits

- Reduces inflammation
- Helps with arthritis and osteoarthritis pain because it's loaded with antioxidants
- Aids the digestive process
- Aids your immune system

- Helps to reduce migraine symptoms
- Helps to reduce nausea and vomiting
- May help with menstrual cramps
- The active ingredients include paradols, gingerols, zingerone, and shogoals; these reduce levels of proinflammatory leukotrienes. Ginger also inhibits the cyclooxygenase enzymes of the inflammatory cascade. Ginger inhibits activation of the proinflammatory nuclear factor kB.

Daily Dosage: 0.5–3 g

Warnings: Ginger may cause side effects such as abdominal discomfort, heartburn, diarrhea, or mouth and throat irritation. Ginger is well known, however, to aid with digestion.

Glutathione

- Naturally present in every cell; it is part of your innate defense against oxidative stress
- Improves levels of protein, enzymes, and bilirubin in those with liver problems
- The main antioxidant defense molecule in the body
- Important in making DNA
- Supports strong immune cell function
- Helps regenerate levels of vitamin C and E
- Cofactor for enzymes involved in fighting free radicals
- Can help to remove some heavy metals from cells

Foods: Strawberries, asparagus, okra, peaches, spinach, avocado, tomatoes

Daily Dosage: 500–2,000 mg daily; 500 mg is typical

Side effects: Skin lightening has been reported; nausea, abdominal bloating, and some have allergic reactions.

Magnesium

Benefits
- Stabilizes the heart rhythm
- Regulates metabolism
- Lowers blood pressure by dilating the arteries
- Relaxes the bronchial tubes, thereby helping with asthma
- Slows aging of cells
- Improves how the immune system responds to invaders[4]
- Supports nerve function and reduces symptoms of restless leg syndrome. It also helps to reduce neuropathic pain.
- Supports bone health and metabolism. Without magnesium, calcium and vitamin D3 cannot function well.

Foods: Whole-grain breads and cereals, spinach, quinoa, soybeans, lima beans, nuts (almonds, cashews, peanuts), avocados, beets, dates, raisins, black beans, dark chocolate

Daily Dosage: 200–400 mg daily. Up to 56 percent of Americans are deficient in magnesium. There are a variety of magnesium salts; some forms have less elemental magnesium than others.

Warnings: Deficiencies are linked to those with type 1 and 2 diabetes, metabolic syndrome, and obesity.[5] Other conditions linked to deficiencies: hypertension, stroke, atherosclerosis, cardiovascular disease, insulin resistance, asthma, chronic fatigue, depression.[6] Deficiencies can also lead to muscle weakness and cramps, insomnia, vomiting, nausea, diarrhea, numbness, tingling seizures, abnormal heart rhythms, erectile dysfunction, and thyroid alterations.[7]

Melatonin

Benefits:
- Reduces inflammation and protects against oxidative stress, highly antioxidant
- Boosts immunity and anticancer activity; antidiabetic and antiaging
- Protects the cardiovascular system
- Protects the neurological system
- May modulate the circadian system and aid sleep
- Melatonin has many properties that support cartilage health and help to control symptoms of arthritis.

Foods: Eggs, salmon, chicken, legumes, yellow corn, nuts (pistachios and walnuts), certain types of mushrooms, cereals, rice, oats, pineapples, tart cherries, grapes, cranberries, kiwis, strawberries, germinated legumes, cauliflower, cucumbers, turnips, tomatoes, peppers

Daily Needs or Dosage: 1–10 mg

Warnings: Melatonin may cause nausea, headache, or dizziness.

NMN–Nicotinamide Mononucleotide

Benefits
- This is a so-called longevity molecule and has been used for many years in the natural medicine community. Vitamin B3 is used to synthesize NMN in the body. NMN is converted to NAD+ (nicotinamide adenine dinucleotide) once consumed. NAD+ confers significant health benefits that can help to improve symptoms of arthritis. NAD+ levels fall in humans with age.

- Provides support to mitochondrial function of cells in joints, connective tissues, muscle, and bone. NAD+ moves electrons to mitochondria for energy production.
- Improves mood and energy levels, increases metabolic rates, and helps to reduce weight gain
- Assists in DNA mutation repair and detoxification of cells through upregulation of sirtuins
- Reduces adipose inflammation, is restorative of muscle, and prevents cognitive decline
- Enhances insulin secretion

Oat Straw Extract

Benefits
- Fights chronic inflammation
- Provides calcium to strengthen bones
- Provides nutrients such as iron, manganese, and zinc
- May relieve stress, anxiety, and depression by inhibiting the enzyme phosphodiesterase type 4, found in immune cells
- May improve brain function by increasing theta electric brain activity in the left frontotemporal region during concentration
- May increase testosterone levels
- May lower cholesterol
- May help with weight reduction

Foods: Oat straw stems and leaves

Daily Needs or Dosage: 800–1,600 mg

Warnings: Side effects may include gas, bloating, and skin irritations.

Omega-3 Fatty Acids

Benefits

- Protects heart by reducing triglycerides and high blood pressure, raises HDL (good) cholesterol levels, prevents blood clots, and prevents plaque in the arteries. Reduces fat in the liver.
- Reduces levels of proinflammatory eicosanoids, cytokines, and cyclo-oxygenase to relieve pain more effectively than NSAIDs. Highly anti-inflammatory and increases levels of resolvins and protectins to promote tissue healing.
- Maintains cell membrane fluidity and function. Provides lubrication to the joints. Improves the flexibility and function of connective tissue cells.
- Maintains nerve membranes and myelin sheath health, supporting neural signaling and keeping neural tissues flexible
- Preserves body composition for patients undergoing chemotherapy and radiation[8]
- Reduces symptoms of depression and anxiety[9]
- Lowers risk of Alzheimer's disease and dementia[10]
- Reduces risk of all-cause mortality, cardiac death, sudden death, and stroke
- Improves bone strength by boosting calcium in bones, thereby reducing the risk of osteoporosis and arthritis
- Reduces the symptoms of arthritis by controlling chronic low-grade inflammation
- Linked to a reduction in risk for macular degeneration and dry eye[11]

Foods: Oily fish (mackerel, anchovies, herring, salmon, tuna, including canned tuna, halibut, sea bass), other seafoods, walnuts, avocados, flaxseeds, flaxseed oil, canola oil, soybeans, chia seeds, algae. Other foods fortified with omega-3s include eggs, margarine, milk, juice, yogurt.

Daily Dosage: 1,000–4,000 mg daily divided between EPA and DHA

Warnings: Deficiencies delay the conversion of light energy to neural energy in the retina. Overdoses of omega-3 can increase the risk of atrial fibrillation, an irregular heart rhythm.[12]

Paprika

Benefits
- Contains capsaicin, a substance found in peppers, which acts as an antioxidant to fight chronic inflammation
- Contains carotenoids and is strongly antioxidant
- Provides calcium, potassium, phosphorus, folate, choline, niacin, vitamin B6, vitamin E, and vitamin K—all important for strong teeth, bones, and muscle
- Improves fat metabolism
- May boost eye health (lowers risk for macular degeneration and cataracts) because of the vitamin E, beta carotene, lutein, and zeaxanthin
- Has analgesic effects for pain management (topical form)
- May improve cholesterol levels (raising HDL)
- May help control blood sugar by inhibiting enzymes that break down sugar in the body
- May have appetite-suppressing properties; can assist with obesity reduction
- May protect skin from UV-induced damage
- Has high levels of carotenoids, which are strong antioxidants

Daily Dosage: No consensus. 20–100 mg daily.

Warnings: Paprika is safe when used in typical cooking amounts, but the spice may cause allergic reactions (skin rash, itching in the mouth, coughing from inhalation, difficulty breathing) in some people.

PEA (Palmitoylethanolamide)

Benefits

- PEA is a common agent to treat nerve-based pain in Europe.
- Fights inflammation, reduces pain, and improves function in people with osteoarthritis
- Binds to cells in the body and may reduce pain and swelling from a number of causes (fibromyalgia, multiple sclerosis, carpal tunnel syndrome)
- PEA is a component of your endocannabinoid system and is important for homeostasis of all other systems; it is produced throughout the body.
- Controls neuropathic pain by reducing the degranulation of mast cells near nerve endings
- Supports brain health and is associated with improved cognition and better mood

Foods: Egg yolks, peanuts

Daily Dosage: 300–1,200 mg

Warnings: PEA is generally safe but may cause nausea in some people.

Potassium

Benefits

- Decreases aging in the arteries
- Carries an electrical charge to help nerve and muscle physiology
- Regulates blood pressure
- Allows the heart and kidneys to function properly

Foods: Avocados, bananas, beans, nuts, dairy, raisins, apricots, potatoes, winter squash, spinach, broccoli, beet greens

Daily Needs or Dosage: 3,000–4,700 mg

Warnings: An overdose of potassium can cause fatigue, weakness, nausea, vomiting, breathing difficulty, chest pain, irregular heartbeats, or numbness and tingling. Potassium deficiencies may lead to many of the same symptoms.

Resveratrol

Benefits

- Acts as a strong antioxidant, associated with increased lifespan and health span
- Induces the production of healthy mitochondria and repairs damaged ones, decreasing the aging of DNA and decreasing the aging of the arteries
- Aids the immune system (antiviral and anticancer effects)
- Protects nerve cells from plaque buildup that leads to Alzheimer's disease
- Helps prevent insulin resistance that leads to diabetes
- Protects the heart by preventing apoptotic cell death in the heart and preventing blood clots. It reduces the oxidation of bad (LDL) cholesterol, thus helping to prevent atherosclerosis.
- Helps heal wounds
- Reduces the pain and inflammation associated with arthritis
- Improves the function of chondrocytes and helps to promote DNA repair through upregulation of sirtuins

Foods: Red grapes, red wine, peanuts, pistachios, berries, cranberries, dark chocolate

Daily Dosage: 500–1,000 mg daily

Warnings: It can interact with blood thinners, blood pressure drugs, cancer treatments, antidepressants, NSAIDs, and other supplements.

Rosemary

Benefits[13]
- The active ingredients are rosmarinic acid, carnosic acid, and carnosol.
- Inhibits some foodborne pathogens (like listeria, B. cereus, and S. aureus)
- May help with indigestion
- May decrease conditions associated with inflammation, acting as a strong antioxidant, neutralizing free radicals. It has also been shown to reduce levels of heterocyclic amines (HCAs) formed by high-temperature meat cooking. It is also known to reduce the risk of oxidation by radiation.
- May alleviate complications of obesity and diabetes
- May reduce muscle pain cause by arthritis. Rosemary is highly anti-inflammatory.
- May assist with neurological deficits and may improve memory and mood.
- May lower cortisol levels and help reduce anxiety
- May stimulate hair growth
- May support the circulatory system

Daily Dosage: 1–4 g daily; there is no consensus.

Warnings: Large doses of rosemary may cause excessive menstrual bleeding and can cause miscarriage. Excessive amounts can result in stomach and intestinal irritation, vomiting, kidney damage, seizures, toxicity, coma, or excess fluid in the lungs.

Saffron

Benefits[14]

- Active ingredients are crocin and safranal.
- Improves symptoms related to depression; enhances mood. The active ingredients increase levels of serotonin, dopamine, and norepinephrine in the brain.
- Improves symptoms related to neurodegenerative conditions and protects from disorders related to the nervous system
- Improves symptoms related to diabetes
- Improves symptoms related to cardiovascular disease
- Saffron is a powerful pain reliever. It reduces levels of inflammatory biomarkers and improves symptoms of people with arthritis.[15]
- Helpful in reducing muscle soreness

Foods: None; saffron is added during food preparation.

Daily Dosage: There is no consensus.

Warnings: Side effects of saffron are rare, but eating too much can be toxic—particularly during pregnancy (5 g is considered a toxic dose). Saffron is very expensive and might cost upward of $10,000 US per pound wholesale.

Schisandra Berry

Benefits

- Works as an adaptogen
- Acts as a super antioxidant, protecting the nerves and helping reduce neuropathic pains
- Improves liver function by reducing the amount of fat in alcohol-induced fatty liver disease

- Relaxes blood vessels due to an increase in an enzyme called endothelial nitric oxide synthase (eNOS), allowing increased blood flow
- Decreases cortisol by 200 percent after exercise. Lower cortisol levels help the body recover faster, build muscle faster, and burn fat better.
- Aids with insomnia, anxiety, depression, and inflammation by lowering cortisol levels
- Improves mental performance in a stressful situation by improved signaling of cell pathways
- Reduces blood glucose levels by inhibition of alpha-glucosidase in the gut, reduces formation of AGEs

Daily Needs or Dosage: 1.5–6 g daily, 500–2,000 mg extract

Warnings: The schisandra berry extract is safe in normal amounts. Side effects include heartburn, upset stomach, decreased appetite, or itching.

Tart Cherry Extract

Benefits
- Active ingredients are anthocyanins, phenols, and flavonoids.
- Reduces inflammation and related pain. Reduces pain by downregulating the cyclooxygenase enzymes, with little or none of the digestive or cardiac side effects associated with NSAIDs.
- Helps reduce symptoms of arthritis and gout (joint pain). Tart cherry extract inhibits the activity of xanthine oxidase in the liver and reduces serum urate levels. It is highly antioxidant and prevents damage by free radicals to cartilage, connective tissue, bone, and muscle.
- Helps improve mitochondrial and cell function because of high antioxidant levels
- May increase muscle strength and reduce muscle soreness after exercise
- Also contains small amounts of melatonin, another powerful antioxidant

Foods: Tart cherries, almonds, chocolate, green tea, pineapples, apples, celery

Daily Dosage: 500 mg–4 g daily

Warnings: To get the same benefits of a daily tart cherry extract supplement, you'd need to eat more than a hundred cherries a day. A cup of cherry juice provides only 60 mg. So getting these benefits through a supplement seems the easier choice, with none of the sugars and fructose associated with juice. Fructose, found in the juice or juice concentrates, will increase levels of urate in the serum.

Turmeric/Curcumin/Quercetin

Benefits[16]
- Reduces inflammation associated with arthritis, helping to relieve pain from joints and connective tissue
- Reduces inflammation in general and symptoms of associated problems
- Helps to rebalance estrogen levels in menopausal women, cooling hot flashes
- Helps with liver disease
- Supports weight control
- Helps with depression
- Aids the immune system
- May help treat diabetes
- May help treat metabolic syndrome

Daily Dosage: 1,200–1,800 mg; usual dose is 1,000 mg curcuminoids.

Warnings: Some recommend against using turmeric if taking Warfarin.

Vitamin A

Benefits
- Supports vision
- Aids the immune system
- Aids the reproductive system
- Helps your heart, lungs, and other organs work functionally
- Essential to human health; deficiency can cause death or blindness
- Beta-carotene is provitamin A, which is a source of retinol.

Foods: Fish, dairy, eggs, organ meats, fruits (including cantaloupe, mangos, apricots) and vegetables (including spinach, sweet potatoes, carrots, broccoli, winter squash)

Daily Needs or Dosage: 700–900 mcg (no higher than 1,500–2,500 IU/day)

Warnings: An overdose has the opposite effect of an antioxidant—it oxidizes tissue, which causes DNA damage and can add to the risk of lung cancer and atherosclerosis. Excess doses can cause fat storage in the liver, chronic hepatitis, and cirrhosis. (Don't concern yourself with getting too much vitamin A through your food.) Most carotenoids are not toxic when taken in excessive amounts, while vitamin A can be. Too much Vitamin A can cause headaches, blurred vision, nausea, dizziness, muscle aches, and coordination problems, and can even lead to coma and death.

Vitamin B1 (Thiamine)

Benefits
- Helps convert food into energy. B1 is a critical cofactor for many processing enzymes.

- Aids in the growth, development, and function of your cells
- Integral to formation of DNA

Foods: Whole grains and fortified bread, cereal, pasta, rice, pork, fish, legumes, including black beans, soybeans, seeds, nuts

Daily Needs or Dosage: 50–100 mg BID or TID

Warnings: Deficiencies are rare in the United States, but certain groups may have trouble getting enough in foods: alcoholics, the elderly, those with HIV/AIDS, diabetics, those who have had bariatric surgery. Subclinical deficiency is quite common.

Vitamin B2 (Riboflavin)

Benefits
- Helps convert food into energy
- Supports the growth, development, and function of your cells

Foods: Eggs, organ meats (kidneys, liver), low-fat milk, mushrooms, spinach, fortified cereals, and grain products

Daily Dosage: 5–10 mg

Warnings: Deficiencies are rare in the United States, but groups that may have trouble getting enough riboflavin include vegetarians, people who don't eat dairy, and pregnant and breastfeeding women and their babies. Deficiencies may cause skin disorders, sores at the corners of your mouth, swollen and cracked lips, hair loss, sore throat, liver disorders, and problems with the reproductive system and nervous system.

Vitamin B3 (Niacin)

Benefits

- Regulates cholesterol. Helps lower bad (LDL) cholesterol and tri-glycerides. Increases good (HDL) cholesterol.
- Reduces the risk of heart attack and stroke in those with atherosclerosis
- Aids in metabolic functions and other growth processes like energy production, cell division, cell replication, and cell growth
- Aids in creating sex hormones and stress-related hormones in the adrenal glands
- Improves insulin sensitivity
- Helps with hair growth
- Improves circulation and blocks fats from being broken down (which reduces the amount of fats in circulation)
- Can cause flushing, and might increase uric acid levels

Foods: Meat, poultry, fish, eggs, green vegetables, nuts, legumes, grains, nutritional yeast

Daily Dosage: 14–30 mg; doses up to 2000 mg have been used to treat hyper-cholesterolemia, but physician monitoring is required.

Warnings: Deficiencies are rare in the United States, but some groups may not get enough niacin in their food: undernourished people with AIDS, alcoholics, anorexics, those with inflammatory bowel disease, cirrhosis, Hartnup disease (a rare genetic disorder), and tumors in their gastrointestinal tract. Deficiencies can lead to rough skin that turns red or brown in the sun, a bright red tongue, vomiting, constipation, or diarrhea, depression, fatigue, blurred vision, high blood sugar, nausea, heartburn, abdominal pain, or aggressive paranoid or suicidal behavior. Subclinical deficiency is quite common.

Vitamin B5 (Pantothenic Acid)

Benefits
- Helps convert food into energy
- Aids in making and breaking down fats during digestion

Foods: Beef, poultry, seafood, organ meats, eggs, milk, mushrooms, avocados, potatoes, broccoli, whole grains (such as whole wheat, brown rice, and oats), peanuts, sunflower seeds, and chickpeas

Daily Dosage: 1–6 mg

Warnings: Deficiencies are rare in the United States, but severe deficiency can cause numbness and burning of the hands and feet, headaches, fatigue, irritability, insomnia, stomach pain, heartburn, diarrhea, nausea, vomiting, and loss of appetite.

Vitamin B6 (Pryridoxine)

Benefits
- Plays a part in more than one hundred enzyme reactions during metabolism
- Depleted with refined carbohydrate diets, HRTs, diuretics
- Coenzyme for metabolism of neurotransmitters, amino acids, conversion of ALA to EPA/DHA
- Reduces incidence and symptoms of trigger fingers, numbness, carpal tunnel syndrome, joint pain
- Decreases homocysteine levels
- Reduces symptoms of PMS, including moodiness, irritability, forgetfulness, bloating, and anxiety

Foods: Poultry, fish, organ meats, starchy vegetables like potatoes; fruit, except citrus

Daily Dosage: 1.3–2 mg can be taken as P5P (pyridoxal 5 phosphate); P5P will not reach toxic levels. 100 mg for thirty days can help one to remember dreams.

Warnings: Deficiencies are rare in the United States, but they can cause anemia, itch, rashes, scaly skin on the lips, cracks at the corner of the mouth, swollen tongue, depression confusion, and a weak immune system. Infants without enough vitamin B6 can develop extremely sensitive hearing or experience seizures.

Vitamin B7 (Biotin)

Benefits
  • Helps turn carbohydrates, fats, and proteins in your food into energy

Foods: Meat, fish, eggs, and organ meats (liver), seeds, nuts, sweet potatoes, spinach, broccoli

Daily Dosage: 3–35 mcg, or 0.003 mg–0.035 mg

Warnings: Deficiencies are uncommon, but these groups may not get enough biotin: alcoholics, pregnant or breastfeeding women, or those with the rare genetic disorder called biotinidase deficiency. Deficiencies can cause thinning hair, rash around the eyes, nose, mouth, or anal area, pinkeye, high levels of acid in the blood and urine, seizures, skin infection, brittle nails, and nervous system disorders.

Vitamin B9 (Folate/Folic Acid)

Benefits
- Folate is the natural form; folic acid is in synthetic form. Folic acid is synthetic and is fully oxidized—it is more stable. Folic acid also has more bioavailability. Conversion of folic acid to active form takes longer with folic acid than with the natural form.
- Reduces homocysteine levels dramatically (elevated homocysteine levels double the risk of stroke)
- Needed for production of DNA and its repair
- Helps cells to divide properly
- May reduce the risk of cancer (but very high doses can increase the risk of colorectal cancer progression)
- Reduces migraine symptoms, improves neurotransmitter levels, protects from anemia

Foods: Salmon, tuna, hamburgers, lamb, beef liver, brussels sprouts, asparagus, spinach, mustard greens, artichokes, black-eyed peas, kidney beans, oranges, sunflower seeds, peanuts, chicken, bananas, tomatoes, bran

Daily Dosage: 400–500 mcg. Methylation genetic issues, MTHFR, might interfere in metabolism.

Warnings: Most people in the United States get enough through foods, but people with disorders that lower nutrient absorption such as those with celiac disease or inflammatory bowel disease may have deficiencies. Folate levels drop dramatically as you age. Subclinical deficiencies are common.

Vitamin B12 (Cobalamin)

Benefits
- Serves in forming red blood cells and in neurological function, assists with myelin formation
- Helps create DNA, RNA, hormones, cholesterol, and neurotransmitters; important in the myelination of nerve fibers
- Helps maintain metabolism by converting food into glucose, then into energy to fight fatigue. Breaks down proteins, fats, and carbohydrates into a more usable form.
- Facilitates cell growth and division
- Delays mental decline and brain atrophy associated with dementia
- Helps prevent anemia
- Aids in the oxidation of odd-chain fatty acids
- Reduces symptoms of diabetic neuropathy

Foods: Fish (clams), poultry, meat (beef liver), dairy, eggs, milk

Daily Dosage: 2.4–2.8 mcg daily per the NIH. Many take 1,000 mcg daily or monthly. There is no consensus on optimal intake—it is dependent upon age, medications, conditions, genetics, and so on. This is a water-soluble vitamin and must be replaced daily.

Warnings: Side effects include constipation and heartburn, but are not common. Deficiencies affect these groups: elderly, diabetics, alcoholics, those who've had bariatric surgery, those on dialysis, those with autoimmune diseases, those with GI diseases, such as celiac or Crohn's. People on metformin, methotrexate, and some other medications may also have a B vitamin deficiency overall. Deficiencies can lead to anemia. Deficiencies can also lead to depression, memory loss, impaired sensory and motor function, and loss of bone density, muscle weakness, migraines, constipation, appetite loss, weight loss, and nerve-based pain syndromes.

Vitamin C (Ascorbic Acid)

Benefits

- Ascorbic acid is a synthetic molecule and is found in vitamin C
- Essential to our diet
- Serves as an essential cofactor to a variety of reactions
- Contributes to immune defense by supporting various cellular functions
- Supports the skin barrier, protecting against pathogens from the environment, and protects from oxidative stress damage due to UV radiation
- This is a potent single-molecule free radical scavenger, antioxidant
- Aids with symptoms of the common cold. Prevents and treats respiratory and systemic infections; it is critical to immune function.
- Lowers the risk of cardiovascular disease, reduces oxidation of LDL
- Decreases tissue damage and is fundamental to the building of collagen. Vital to connective tissue health.
- Prevents bone loss associated with osteoporosis and cartilage insufficiencies linked to aging
- May slow the progression of macular degeneration of the eyes
- Supports wound healing

Daily Dosage: 1,000 mg/day up to 6,000 mg/day, but there is no consensus. This is a water-soluble vitamin and must be replaced daily. IV treatments increase plasma concentrations much more than oral dosing. RDAs are much lower. 2,000 mg daily can cause digestive discomfort. Up to 10,000 mg per day has shown no adverse effects. Higher doses have some association with kidney stones and uric acid formation.

Warnings: Deficiency impairs immunity and increases risks of infections. Groups who may tend to have deficiencies include smokers, those exposed to secondhand smoke, those with kidney disease requiring dialysis, infants who are fed evaporated or boiled cow's milk, people who eat a very limited variety of food, or those with medical conditions that prevent them from absorbing vitamin C. Alcohol reduces vitamin C levels as well.

Vitamin D

Benefits
- A hormone that is produced in the skin at levels of up to 25,000 IUs every day normally. Deficiencies result from a lack of sun exposure or lack of provitamin D3 in the diet.
- Increases the absorption of calcium, vital for healthy bones, muscle, nerves, and intercellular communications
- Slows the progression of osteoarthritis, strengthening muscles, joints, and bones so they move properly
- Helps manage osteopenia and osteoporosis
- Regulates blood sugar
- Protects against cardiovascular disease, reducing cholesterol levels and high blood pressure; deficiency associated with congestive heart failure
- Aids your nervous system in carrying messages between your brain and body
- Aids in metabolism
- Aids your immune system to fight off invading bacteria and viruses
- Reduces your risk for depression and enhances brain and immune function
- Associated with reduced symptoms in MS

Foods: Oily fish (trout, salmon, tuna, mackerel), shellfish, beef liver, eggs, cheese, fortified milk, soy milk, almond milk, oat milk, orange juice, fortified cereals, mushrooms

Daily Dosage: There is no consensus; optimal health requires higher levels than the RDA in my opinion. Older women need more than younger men.

Athletes need more than nonathletes. Everyone needs optimal levels to prevent multiple health problems. The range is 100 IU to 5000 IU daily. If deficiency is present, even higher doses are usually prescribed. Long-term high dose supplementation has been shown safe. Blood levels should stay below 150 ng/dL to prevent toxicity.

Warnings: Deficiency increases pain from arthritis and causes your bones to become fragile. Deficiencies are more likely in these groups: breastfed babies, the elderly, those who have limited exposure to sunlight, people with dark skin, people with conditions that limit fat absorption (Crohn's, celiac, ulcerative colitis), people who are obese or those who've had gastric bypass surgery. An overdose can lead to nausea, vomiting, muscle weakness, confusion, pain, dehydration, excessive urination/thirst, and kidney stones.

Vitamin E

Benefits
- Acts as an antioxidant to protect cells from the damage caused by free radicals; it is fat-soluble and prevents oxidation of cell membranes, prevents damage to PUFAs in the membrane. Alpha-tocopherol is the preferred form.
- Boosts the innate immune system to fight off invading bacteria and viruses
- Shown to have cardiovascular benefits and is neuroprotective
- Supports liver cells in the setting of NAFLD (nonalcoholic fatty-liver disease)
- Vitamin E is highly anti-inflammatory.

Foods: Vegetable oils (wheat germ, sunflower, safflower, corn, soybean), peanuts, hazelnuts, almonds, sunflower seeds, green vegetables (spinach, broccoli), fortified cereals

Daily Dosage: 15–19 mg

Warnings: Deficiencies are rare in healthy people. A deficiency is almost always linked to diseases that limit absorption (Crohn's disease, cystic fibrosis, and rare genetic diseases). Deficiencies can result in nerve and muscle damage that lead to a loss of feeling in the arms and legs, loss of control of movement, muscle weakness, vision problems, and a weakened immune system. Subclinical deficiencies are common due to limited dietary intake.

Vitamin K

Benefits

- Aids in blood clotting, inhibits vessel-wall calcifications, supports endothelial integrity
- Strengthens bones, facilitating mineralization and calcium homeostasis
- Involved in tissue renewal and cell growth
- May prevent heart disease by making blood vessels that lead to the heart less stiff and narrow
- Involved in the production and regulation of osteocalcin, along with vitamin D
- Osteocalcin can improve insulin sensitivity
- Shown to reduce the incidence of hip fractures, improves bone density
- Enhances the ability of bisphosphonates to support bone health in osteoporosis (45 mg K2 daily)

Foods: Leafy vegetables (spinach, kale, broccoli, lettuce), vegetable oils, some fruits (blueberries, figs), meat, cheese, eggs, soybeans, alfalfa

Daily Dosage: 45–700 mcg (MK4, MK7)

Warnings: Deficiencies are very rare, but certain groups may experience a deficiency: newborns who don't receive an injection at birth, those who have cystic fibrosis, celiac disease, ulcerative colitis, and short bowel syndrome, and those who've had bariatric surgery. Subclinical deficiency seems to be common. Side effects are rare, but it can interfere with certain medications like warfarin. Warfarin is a vitamin K antagonist.

Zinc

Benefits

- Is essential for your immune system to function[17]
- Is an anti-inflammatory, reducing cytokines and oxidative stress[18]
- Reduces the risk for the common cold and speeds recovery
- Helps prevent blindness in patients with age-related dry type of macular degeneration[19]
- Helps the body make proteins, DNA, and genetic materials in all the cells. Zinc is a cofactor for hundreds of chemical reactions in the body.
- Helps wounds heal; slowly healing wounds are a sign of deficiency.
- Is essential for the proper senses of taste and smell
- Provides assistance with the metabolism of alcohol
- Intake of zinc should be balanced with appropriate levels of copper

Foods: Pulses and cereals, along with animal proteins such as red meats and oysters

Daily Dosage: 11–13 mg elemental; with a salt added, such as zinc gluconate, the range increases to 100–400 mg daily.

Warnings: Deficiency leads to increased infections. Certain groups are more prone to deficiencies: those with digestive disorders (Crohn's, celiac, ulcerative colitis), vegetarians, alcoholics, and those with sickle cell disease. Those with low levels of zinc have a greater risk of pneumonia and other infections. Overdoses of zinc can cause nausea, vomiting, stomach cramps, diarrhea, and headaches. Zinc can interfere with other medications such as antibiotics, penicillamine, and some diuretics. Zinc may be toxic in higher doses and is linked to copper deficiencies.

APPENDIX II

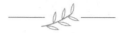

SUPPLEMENTS BY HEALTH CONDITION

Osteoarthritis

- Glucosamine
- Glutathione
- Chondroitin
- Omega-3
- Resveratrol
- PEA
- Vitamin C
- Vitamin E
- Alpha-Lipoic Acid
- Turmeric
- Schisandra Berry
- Ginger
- Turmeric
- Black Pepper
- Tart Cherry
- Delta 8

Muscle Weakness, Fatigue, Pain

- Tart Cherry Extract
- CoQ10
- Creatine
- Alcar
- Glutathione
- Turmeric
- Piperine
- Omega 3
- Ginseng
- B Vitamins
- PEA
- Alpha-Lipoic Acid
- CBD
- Saffron

Nerve Pain

- Alpha-Lipoic Acid
- PEA
- Resveratrol
- Luteolin
- Omega 3
- NAC (N-Acetyl L-Cysteine)
- Vitamin B Complex
- Delta 8
- PEA
- GABA
- Vitamin D3

Brain Support

- Acetyl-L-Carnitine
- Caffeine
- L-Tyrosine
- Choline
- Chaga
- Cordyceps
- Lion's Mane
- Reishi
- Noopept
- Bacopa Monnieri
- Phosphatidylserine

Longevity Support

- Berberine
- NMN
- Resveratrol
- Quercetin
- Glutathione
- Cysteine
- N-Acetyl-Cysteine

Weight Loss and Glucose Management

- L-Carnitine
- Chromium Chloride
- Berberine
- ALA

Sample Patient Profile and Recommendation

Let's say that Bill presents with complaints of restless leg syndrome, stiffness, and burning foot pain. After a thorough workup, I would recommend ALA in the morning, and PEA at night. If he can do it, I would add tart cherry extract at night as well. Delta8 THC is extremely helpful for neuropathic pain, particularly the topical version for areas like the hands, feet, elbows, shoulders, and knees. For his stiffness, the best I have found is omega-3. Depending upon the success of this regimen, which will take two to three months to take effect, I may add NMN and resveratrol in the morning with a fatty food/drink.

Now, if Jane comes in and she simply has knee osteoarthritis or something similar, the group of supplements I find the most effective is curcuminoids with ginger and PEA and then tart cherry extract. Omega-3 capsules are extremely helpful in reducing her pain and stiffness. In addition, omega-3 has the added benefit of reducing brain inflammation and assisting mood.

For my postoperative patients, for many years I have recommended calcium, zinc, vitamin C, magnesium, and vitamin D3. Given the number of supplements involved, the very first product I made for my natural medicine line was one that incorporated all of these into a single bottle. That supplement created the Well Theory—my line of natural products to help optimize your health—and was much easier on my patients. Today, this group of vitamins and minerals, which all improve the immune system and, thus, healing from a surgery, will include either PEA or CBD to help reduce the inflammatory pain of surgery.

If you are wondering what supplements might help you to harness the power of your mind in your quest for a health mindset, here are my favorites. All of these work to reduce inflammation in the brain, decreasing negativity, irritability, and brain fog. They will also help to improve balance and ability of neurons and to increase the ability of your executive function to regulate the amygdala.

- Omega 3
- Tryptophan
- 5-HT Alcar
- L-Tyrosine
- Oat Straw Extract
- PEA

Also, lion's mane, chaga, and cordyceps are great mushroom-sourced supplements that provide excellent outcomes with regard to brain function.

ACKNOWLEDGMENTS

I am profoundly grateful to my family and clinical staff for their enduring support and understanding as I worked on this book. This has been a labor of love and a true passion of mine for some time. Their patience and encouragement kept me grounded. I wish to express my sincere appreciation to the wonderfully talented team at BenBella, especially my editors Gregory Newton Brown and Claire Schulz. It has been a true privilege to work with such a gifted team so devoted to empowering readers to take charge of their health. I also wish to thank the entire editorial and production staff for their flexibility with my schedule and valuable feedback that refined the manuscript. I would also like to thank Natalie Noel, without whom this book would not have been possible. She has a tireless dedication to my vision of educating the public on health and wellness. Without Natalie's contributions, I could not have produced a book that makes complex health concepts understandable and actionable for readers. The partnership with her and with BenBella has been essential to fulfilling my mission of empowering you, the reader, with the knowledge you need to understand and optimize your own health and wellness.

NOTES

CHAPTER ONE: WHY THE WELL THEORY

1. Bridget M. Kuehn, "US Health System Ranks Last Among High-Income Countries," *JAMA* 326, no. 11 (2021): 999, https://doi.org/10.1001/jama.2021.15468.

2. John Poisal et al., "National Health Expenditure Projections, 2021–2030: Growth to Moderate As Covid Impacts Wane," *Health Affairs* 41, no. 4 (March 2022), https://doi.org/10.1377/hlthaff.2022.00113.

3. S. Samuel Bederman et al., "Who's in the Driver's Seat? The Influence of Patient and Physician Enthusiasm on Regional Variation in Degenerative Lumbar Surgery," *Spine* 36, no. 6: 481–489, https://doi.org/10.1097/brs.0b013e3181d25e6f; S. R. Lopushinsky et al., "Regional Variation in Surgery for Gastroesophageal Reflux Disease in Ontario," *Surgical Innovation* 14, no. 1 (2007): 35–40, https://doi.org/10.1177/1553350606298967; James N. Weinstein et al., "Surgical Versus Nonsurgical Therapy for Lumbar Spinal Stenosis" (in all, more than thirty-five studies are listed in the references section of this article), *The New England Journal of Medicine* 358, no. 8 (2008): 794–810, https://doi.org/10.1056/NEJMoa0707136.

4. S. Samuel Bederman, "Who's in the Driver's Seat? The Influence of Patient and Physician Enthusiasm on Regional Variation in Degenerative Lumbar Spinal Surgery," *Spine* 36, no. 6: 481–489, https://doi.org/10.1097/brs.0b013e3181d25e6f; Micheal Radd et al., "US Regional Variations in Rates, Outcomes, and Costs of Spinal Arthrodesis for Lumbar Spinal Stenosis

in Working Adults Aged 40–65," *Journal of Neurosurgery Spine* 30 (January 2019): 83–90, https://doi.org/10.3171/2018.5.SPINE18184; J. Desai Rishi, "Association of Geography and Access to Healthcare Providers with Long-term Prescription opioid use in Medicare Patients with Severe Osteoarthritis: A Cohort Study," *HHS Public Access* 71, no. 5 (May 2019): 712–721, https://doi .org/10.1002/art.40834; Elliott S. Wennberg et al., "Geography and the Debate Over Medicare Reform," *Medicare* (July 2011): https://doi.org/10.1377/hlthaff .w2.96; Alosh Hassan et al., "Insurance Status, Geography, Race, and Eth-nicity as Predictors of Anterior Cervical Spine Surgery Rates and In-Hospital Mortality," *Spine* 34, no. 18 (2019): 1956–1962, https://doi.org/10.1097 /BRS.0b013e3181ab930e; Janna Friedly et al., "Geographic Variation in Epi-dural Steroid Injection Use in Medicare Patients," *Journal of Bone and Joint Surgery* 90 (2008): 1730–1737, https://doi.org/10.2106/JBJS.G.00858.

5. James N. Weinstein et al., "Trends and Geographic Variations in Major Sur-gery for Degenerative Diseases of the Hip, Knee, and Spine," *Health Affairs* 81, no. 9 (2004): https://doi:10.1377/hlthaff.var.81.

6. I have used the acronym MEDS for many years in my practice. Similar for-mulations have also been used by author Nicholas Bate, physical therapist Dr. Timothy Flynn, and author Brooke McAlary, among others.

7. "Arthritis," CDC, last modified October 5, 2023, https://www.cdc.gov /chronicdisease/resources/publications/factsheets/arthritis.htm.

8. Ruben Castaneda, "OTC Products: How Much Is Too Much?" *U.S. News and World Reports*, June 13, 2017, https://health.usnews.com/wellness/articles /2017-06-13/otc-products-how-much-is-too-much.

9. Adam G. Culvenor et al., "Prevalence of Knee Osteoarthritis Features on Magnetic Resonance Imaging in Asymptomatic Uninjured Adults: A Sys-tem Review and Meta-analysis," *British Journal of Sports Medicine* 53, (2019): 1268–1278, http://dx.doi.org/10.1136/bjsports-2018-099257. This review article lists more than ninety-six similar studies in its References section.

10. David C. Levin et al., "Ownership or Leasing of MRI Facilities by Nonra-diologist Physicians Is a Rapidly Growing Trend," *Journal of the American College of Radiology* 5, no. 2 (2008): 105–09.

11. John Temple, *American Pain: How a Young Felon and His Ring of Doctors Unleashed America's Deadliest Drug Epidemic*, First Lyons Press (2015).

12. Scott D. Boden et al, "Abnormal Magnetic-Resonance Scans of the Lumbar Spine in Asymptomatic Subjects," *The Journal of Bone and Joint Surgery* 72A, no. (March 1990): 403–408.

13. David Borenstein et al., "The Value of Magnetic Resonance Imaging of the Lumbar Spine to Predict Low-Back Pain in Asymptomatic Subjects: A Seven-Year Follow-Up Study," *The Journal of Bone and Joint Surgery* 83A, no. 9 (September 2001): 1306–1311, https://doi.org/10.2106/00004623 -200109000-00002; F. Alyas, M. Turner, and D. Connell, "MRI Findings in the Lumbar Spines of Asymptomatic Adolescent, Elite Tennis Players," *British Journal of Sports Medicine* 41 (2007): 836–841, https://doi.org/10.1136 /bjsm.2007.037747; Morio Matsumoto et al., "MRI of Cervical Intervertebral Discs in Asymptomatic Subjects," *The Journal of Bone & Joint Surgery* 80B, no. 1 (January 1998): 19–24, https://doi.org/10.1302/0301-620x.80b1.7929; Scott D. Boden et al., "Abnormal Magnetic-Resonance Scans of the Lumbar Spine in Asymptomatic Subjects," *The Journal of Bone and Joint Surgery* 72A, no. 3 (March 1990): 403–408; Tapio Videman et al., "Associations Between Back Pain History and Lumbar MRI Findings," *Spine* 28, no. 6 (2003): 582– 588, https://doi.org/10.1097/01.BRS.0000049905.44466.73; Philip McNee et al., "Predictors of Long-Term Pain and Disability in Patients with Low Back Pain Investigated by Magnetic Resonance Imaging: A Longitudinal Study," *BMC Musculoskeletal Disorders* 12, no. 1 (2011): 1–12, https://doi.org /10.1186/1471-2474-12-234.

14. Tiffany K. Gill et al., "Prevalence of Abnormalities on Shoulder MRI in Symptomatic and Asymptomatic Older Adults," *International Journal of Rheumatic Diseases* 17, no. 8 (2014): 863–871, https://doi.org/10.1111/1756-185x.12476; Sari M. Siivola et al., "MRI Changes of Cervical Spine in Asymptomatic and Symptomatic Young Adults," *Europe Spine Journal* 11 (2002): 358– 363, https://doi.org/10.1007/s00586-001-0370-X; Anthony Miniaci et al., "Magnetic Resonance Imaging Evaluation of the Rotator Cuff Tendons in the Asymptomatic Shoulder," *American Journal of Sports Medicine* 23, no. 2 (1995): 142–145, https://doi.org/10.1177/036354659502300202; Patrick M. Connor et al., "Magnetic Resonance Imaging of the Asymptomatic Shoulder of Overhead Athletes: A 5-Year Follow-Up Study," *The American Journal of Sports Medicine* 31, no. 5 (2003): 724–727, https://doi.org

/10.1177/03635465030310051501; Jerry S. Sher et al., "Abnormal Findings on Magnetic Resonance Images of Asymptomatic Shoulders," *JBJS* 77, no. 1 (1995): 10–15, https://doi.org/10.2106/00004623-199501000-00002; Ayane Rossano et al., "Prevalence of Acromioclavicular Joint Osteoarthritis in People Not Seeking Care: A Systematic Review," *Journal of Orthopaedics* 32 (2022): 85–91, https://doi.org/10.1016/j.jor .2022.05.009.

15. Adam G. Culvenor et al., "Prevalence of Knee Osteoarthritis Features on Magnetic Resonance Imagining in Asymptomatic Uninjured Adults: A Systematic Review and Meta-Analysis," *British Journal of Sports Medicine* 53 (2019): 1268–1278, https://doi.org/:10.1136/bjsports-2018-099257; Lee D. Kaplan et al., "Magnetic Resonance Imaging of the Knee in Asymptomatic Professional Basketball Players," *Journal of Arthroscopic and Related Surgery* 21, no. 5 (May 2005): 557–561, https://doi.org/10.1016/j.arthro.2005.01.009; K. A. Beattle et al., "Abnormalities Identified in the Knees of Asymptomatic Volunteers Using Peripheral Magnetic Resonance Imaging," *OsteoArthritis and Cartilage* 13 (2005): 181–186, https://doi.org/10.1016/j.joca.2004.11.001; Marco Zanetti et al., "Patients with Suspected Meniscal Tears: Prevalence of Abnormalities Seen on MRI of 100 Symptomatic and 100 Contralateral Asymptomatic Knees," *American Journal of Roentgenology* 181 (September 2003): 635–641, https://doi.org/0361-803X/03/1813-635.

16. M. Lohman et al., "MRI Abnormalities of Foot and Ankle in Asymptomatic, Physically Active Individuals," *Skeletal Radiology* 30 (2001): 61–66; Robert A. Gallo et al., "Asymptomatic Hip/Groin Pathology Identified on Magnetic Resonance Imaging of Professional Hockey Players: Outcomes and Playing Status at 4 Years' Follow-Up," *Arthroscopy: The Journal of Arthroscopic & Related Surgery* 30, no. 10 (2014): 1222–1228, https:// doi.org/10.1016/j.arthro.2014.04.100; Brad Register et al., "Prevalence of Abnormal Hip Findings in Asymptomatic Participants: A Prospective, Blinded Study," *American Journal of Sports Medicine* 40, no. 12 (2012): 2720–2724, https://doi.org/10.1177/0363546512462124; Florian Tresch et al., "Hip MRI: Prevalence of Articular Cartilage Defects and Labral Tears in Asymptomatic Volunteers: A Comparison with a Matched Population of Patients with Femoroacetabular Impingement," *Journal of Magnetic*

Resonance Imaging 46, no. 2 (2017): 440–451, https://doi.org/10.1002/jmri.25565.

17. Kanu Okike et al., "Accuracy of Conflict-of-Interest Disclosures Reported by Physicians," *New England Journal of Medicine* 361 (2009): 1466–1474, https://doi.org/10.1056/NEJMsa0807160.

18. Okike et al., "Accuracy of Conflict-of-Interest Disclosures Reported by Physicians."

19. Charles Piller, "Blots on a Field," *Science* 377, no. 6604 (July 2022): https://doi.org/1126/Science.ade0209.

20. Anahad O'Connor, "How the Sugar Industry Shifted Blame to Fat," *The New York Times*, September 12, 2016.

21. Joanna Moncrieff et al., "The Serotonin Theory of Depression: A Systematic Umbrella Review of the Evidence," *Molecular Psychiatry* (July 2022): https://doi.org/10.1038/s41380-022-01661-0.

22. Eugene J. Carragee et al., "A Challenge to Integrity in Spine Publications: Years of Living Dangerously with the Promotion of Bone Growth Factors," *The Spine Journal* 11 (2011): 463–468, https://doi.org/10.1016/j.spinee.2011.06.001; Eugene J. Carragee et al, "A Critical Review of Recombinant Human Bone Morphogenetic Protein-2 Trials in Spinal Surgery: Emerging Safety Concerns and Lessons Learned," *The Spine Journal* 11 (2011): 471–491, https://doi.org/10.1016/j.spinee.2011.04.023.

23. Dylan Tanzer et al., "American Academy of Orthopaedic Surgeons Disclosure Policy Fails to Accurately Inform Its Members of Potential Conflicts of Interest," *American Journal of Orthopedics* E (July 2015): 207–211.

24. Gail Chimonas et al., "From Disclosure to Transparency: The Use of Company Payment Data," *Archives of Internal Medicine* 171, no. 1 (2011): 81–86, https://doi.org/10.1001/archinternmed.2010.341.

25. Pauline Anderson, "Doctors' Suicide Rate Highest of Any Profession," *WebMD*, May 8, 2018, https://www.webmd.com/mental-health/news/20180508/doctors-suicide-rate-highest-of-any-profession.

26. O. J. Wouters, "Lobbying Expenditures and Campaign Contributions by the Pharmaceutical and Health Product Industry in the United States, 1999–2018," *JAMA Internal Medicine* (2020): https://doi.org/10.1001/jamainternmed.2020.0146.

27. Eric G. Campbell et al., "A National Survey of Physician-Industry Relationships," *New England Journal of Medicine* 356, no. 17 (2007): 1742–1750, https://doi.org/10.1056/NEJMsa064508.

28. Robert Langreth, "Drug Prices," *Bloomberg*, September 16, 2020, https://www.bloomberg.com/quicktake/drug-prices.

29. Rory J. Ferguson et al., "Hip Replacement," *Lancet* 392, no. 10158 (2018): 1662–1671, https://doi.org/10.1016/S0140-6736(18)31777-X.

30. J. S. Bahl et al., "Changes in 24-Hour Physical Activity Patterns and Walking Gait Biomechanics After Primary Total Hip Arthroplasty: A 2-Year Follow-up Study," *Journal of Bone Joint Surgery of America* 103, no. 13 (July 2021): 1166–1174, https://doi.org/10.2106/JBJS.20.01679.

31. Asbjorn Hrobjartsson and Peter C. Gotzsche, "Is the Placebo Powerless? An Analysis of Clinical Trials Comparing Placebo with No Treatment," *New England Journal of Medicine* 344, no. 21 (May 2001): 1594–1601, https://doi.org/10.1056/NEJM200105243442106.

32. Adriaan Louw et al., "Sham Surgery in Orthopedics: A Systemic Review of the Literature," *Pain Medicine* 18 (2017): 736–750, https://doi.org/10.1093/pm/pnw/164.

CHAPTER TWO: WHY YOUR BODY LOVES ANTIOXIDANTS AND HATES CHRONIC INFLAMMATION

1. Julia B. Ewaschuk et al., "Role of N-3 Fatty Acids in Muscle Loss and Myosteatosis," *Applied Physiology Nutrition & Metabolism* 39 (2014): 1–9, https://doi.org/10.1139/apnm-2013-0423.

2. William S. Harris and Clemens von Schacky, "The Omega-3 Index: A New Risk Factor for Death from Coronary Heart Disease?" *Preventive Medicine* 39, no. 1 (July 2004): 212–220, https://doi.org/10.1016/j.ypmed.2004.02.030.

3. A. J. Bailey, N. D. Light, and Ed Atkins, "Chemical Cross-Linking Restrictions on Models for the Molecular Organization of the Collagen Fiber," *Nature* 288 (November 1980): 408–410, https://doi.org/10.1038/288408a0.

4. Monica H. Carlsen et al., "The Total Antioxidant Content of More Than 3100 Foods, Beverages, Spices, Herbs and Supplements Used Worldwide," *Nutrition Journal* 9, no. 3 (2010): https://doi.org/10.1186/1475-2891-9-3.

5. R. J. Widmer et al., "The Mediterranean Diet, Its Components, and Cardio-vascular Disease," *American Journal of Medicine* 128, no. 3 (2015): 229–238, https://doi.org/10.1016/j.amjmed.2014.10.014.

6. Ramon Estruch, et al., "Primary Prevention of Cardiovascular Disease With a Mediterranean Diet Supplemented with Extra-Virgin Olive Oil or Nuts," *New England Journal of Medicine* 378E, no. 34 (June 2018): https://doi .org/10/1056/NEJMoa1800389.

7. L. Schwingshackl et al., "Adherence to Mediterranean Diet and Risk of Can-cer: An Updated Systematic Review and Meta-Analysis of Observational Studies," *Cancer Medicine* 4, no. 12 (2015): 1933–1947, https://doi.org/10 .1002/cam4.539.

8. F. Sofi et al., "Mediterranean Diet and Health Status: An Updated Meta-Analysis and a Proposal for a Literature-Based Adherence Score," *Pub-lic Health Nutrition* 4, no. 17 (2014): 2769–2782, https://doi.org/10.1017 /S1368980013003169.

9. C. Valls-Pedret et al., "Mediterranean Diet and Age-Related Cognitive Decline: A Randomized Clinical Trial," *JAMA Intern Med* 175, no. 7 (2015): 1094–1103, https://doi.org/10.1001/jamainternmed.2015.1668.

10. K. Esposito et al., "A Journey into a Mediterranean Diet and Type 2 Diabe-tes: A Systematic Review with Meta-Analyses," *British Medical Journal Open* 5, no. 8 (2015): https://doi.org/10.1136/bmjopen-2015-008222.

11. K. Esposito et al., "Mediterranean Diet and Weight Loss: Meta-Analysis of Randomized Controlled Trials," *Metabolic Syndrome and Related Disorders* 9, no. 11 (2011): 1–12, https://doi.org/10.1089/met.2010.0031.

12. T. Colin Campbell and Thomas M. Campbell, *The China Study: The Most Com-prehensive Study of Nutrition Ever Conducted and the Startling Implications for Diet, Weight Loss, and Long-Term Health* (Dallas, BenBella Books, Inc., 2006).

13. D. Buettner and S. Skemp, "Blue Zones: Lessons From the World's Longest Lived," *American Journal of Lifestyle Medicine* 10, no. 5 (July 2016): 318–321, https://doi.org/10.1177/1559827616637066.

14. Dan Buettner, *The Blue Zones Solution: Eating and Living Like the World's Healthiest People* (California: Disney Publishing Group, 2017).

15. Melisa Bailey and Hannah D. Holscher, "Microbiome-Mediated Effects of the Mediterranean Diet on Inflammation," *American Society for Nutrition* 9 (2018): 193–206, https://doi.org/10/1093/advances/nmy013.

16. Pirkko J. Pussinen et al., "Endotoxemia Is Associated with an Increased Risk of Incident Diabetes," *Diabetes Care* 34 (February 2011): 392–395, https://doi.org/10.2337/dc10-1676.

17. Shireen Mohammad and Christoph Thiemermann, "Role of Metabolic Endotoxemia in Systemic Inflammation and Potential Interventions," *Frontiers in Immunology* 11, no. 594150 (January 2021): https://doi.org/10.3389/fimmu.2020.594150.

CHAPTER THREE: THE RADICAL POWER OF A POSITIVE MINDSET

1. A. Steptoe et al., "Positive Affect and Psychobiological Processes Relevant to Health," *Journal of Personality* 77, no. 6 (2009): 1747–1776, https://doi.org/10.1111/j.1467-6494.2009.00599.x.

2. S. Kamping et al., "Deficient Modulation of Pain by a Positive Emotional Context in Fibromyalgia Patients," *Pain* 154, no. 9 (2013): 1846–1855, https://doi.org/10.1016/j.pain.2013.06.003.

3. Patricia H. Rosenberger, Peter Jokl, and Jeannette Ickovics, "Psychosocial Factors and Surgical Outcomes: An Evidence-Based Literature Review," *Journal of the American Academy of Orthopedic Surgeons* 14, no. 7 (July 2006): 397–405, https://doi.org/10.5435/00124635-200607000-00002.

4. David C. Flanigan et al., "Psychological Factors Affecting Rehabilitation and Outcomes Following Elective Orthopaedic Surgery," *Journal of the American Academy of Orthopaedic Surgeons* 23, no 9 (September 2015): 563–570, http://dx.doi.org/10.5435/JAAOS-D-14-00225; Daniel L. Riddle et al., "Preoperative Pain Catastrophizing Predicts Pain Outcome After Knee Arthroplasty," *Clinical Orthopaedics and Related Research* 468 (2010): 798–806, https://doi.org/10.1007/s11999-009-0963-y; Richard L. Skolasky et al., "The

Relationship Between Pain and Depressive Symptoms After Lumbar Spine Surgery," *Journal of Pain* 153, no 10 (October 2012): 2092–2096, https://doi .org/10.106/j.pain.2012.06.026; J. A. Singh et al., "Pessimistic Explanatory Style: A Psychological Risk Factor for Poor Pain and Functional Outcomes Two Years After Knee Replacement," *Journal of Bone & Joint Surgery* 92B (2010): 799–806, https://doi.org/10.1302/0301-620X.92B6.23114; Vikki Wylde et al., "The Role of Preoperative Self-Efficacy in Predicting Outcome After Total Knee Replacement," *Musculoskeletal Care* 10 (2012): 110–118, https://doi.org/10.1002/msc.1008; Maaike Leeuw et al., "The Fear-Avoidance Model of Musculoskeletal Pain: Current State of Scientific Evidence," *Journal of Behavioral Medicine* 30, no. 1 (February 2007): https://doi.org/ 10.1007/ s10865-006-9085-0; Johan W. S. Vlaeyen and Steven J. Linton, "Fear-Avoidance Model of Chronic Musculoskeletal Pain: 12 Years On," *Journal of Pain (International Association for the Study of Pain)* 153 (2012): 1144–1147, https://doi.org/10.1016/j.pain.2011.12.009.

5. D. C. Ayers et al., "The Role of Emotional Health in Functional Outcomes After Orthopaedic Surgery: Extending the Biopsychosocial Model to Orthopaedics," *JBJS-A* 165E (2013): 1–7, http://dx.doi.org/10.2016/JBJS.L.00799.

6. P. M. Trief et al., "Emotional Health Predicts Pain and Function After Fusion: A Prospective Multicenter Study," *Spine* 31, no. 7 (April 2006): 823–830, https://doi.org/10.1097/01.brs.0000206362.03950.5b.

7. R. E. Anakwe et al., "Predicting Dissatisfaction After Total Hip Arthroplasty: A Study of 850 Patients," *Journal of Arthroplasty* 26, no. 2 (February 2011): 209–213, https://doi.org/10.1016/j.arth.2010.03.013.

8. D. A. Heck et al., "Patient Outcomes After Knee Replacement," *Clinical Orthopaedics and Related Research* 356 (November 1998): 93–110, https://doi .org/10.1097/00003086-199811000-00015.

9. A. J. Crum and E. J. Langer, "Mind-Set Matters: Exercise and the Placebo Effect," *Psychological Science* 18, no. 2 (2007): 165–171, https://doi.org /10.1111/j.1467-9280.2007.01867.x.

10. D. J. Lanska and J. T. Lanska, "Franz Anton Mesmer and the Rise and Fall of Animal Magnetism: Dramatic Cures, Controversy, and Ultimately a Triumph for the Scientific Method," In *Brain, Mind and*

Medicine: Essays in Eighteenth-Century Neuroscience: 301–321, https:doi.org/10.1007/978-0-387-70967-3_22.

11. F. Benedetti et al., "The Biochemical and Neuroendocrine Bases of the Hyperalgesic Nocebo Effect," *The Journal of Neuroscience* 26, no. 46 (2006): 12014–12022, https://doi.org/10.1523/JNEUROSCI.2947-06.2006.

12. Ian Harris, *Surgery, The Ultimate Placebo* (Alabama: NewSouth Books, 2016).

13. R. Sihvonen et al., "FIDELITY (Finnish Degenerative Meniscus Lesion Study) Investigators. Arthroscopic Partial Meniscectomy for a Degenerative Meniscus Tear: A 5 Year Follow-Up of the Placebo-Surgery Controlled FIDELITY Trial," *British Journal of Sports Med* 54, no. 22 (2020): 1332–1339, https://doi.org/10.1136/bjsports-2020-102813.

14. B. Hallstrom and R. Meremikwu, "Arthroscopic Treatment of Degenerative Meniscal Tears and Sham Surgery or Physical Therapy–An Update on the ESCAPE Trial," *JAMA Net Open* 5, no.7 (2022): https://doi.org/10.1001/jamanetworkopen.2022.20405.

15. K. R. Sochacki et al., "Sham Surgery Studies in Orthopaedic Surgery May Just Be a Sham: A Systematic Review of Randomized Placebo-Controlled Trials," *Arthroscopy* 26, no. 10 (2020): 1–13, https://doi.org/10.1016/j.arthro.2020.05.001.

16. J. W. Orchard, "Pay Attention to the Evidence: In the Longer Term, Intraarticular Corticosteroid Injections Offer Only Harm for Knee Osteoarthritis," *Osteoarthritis and Cartilage* 31, no. 2 (2023): 142–143, https://doi.org/10.1016/j.joca.2022.10.012.

17. Timothy E. Mcalindon et al., "Effect of Intra-Articular Triamcinolone vs. Saline on Knee Cartilage Volume and Pain in Patients with Knee Osteoarthritis: A Randomized Clinical Trial," *JAMA* 317, no. 19 (2017): 1967–1975, https://doi.org/10.1001/jama.2017.5283.

18. A. Jinich-Diamant et al., "Neurophysiological Mechanisms Supporting Mindfulness Meditation-Based Pain Relief: An Updated Review," *Current Pain and Headache Reports* 24, no. 10 (2020): 1–10, https://doi.org/10.1007/s11916-020-00890-8.

19. A. K. Resenstiel and F. J. Keefe, "The Use of Coping Strategies in Chronic Low Back Pain Patients: Relationship to Patient Characteristics and Current Adjustment," *Pain* 17, no. 1 (1983): 33–44, https://doi.org/10.1016/0304 -3959(83)90125-2; M. J. L. Sullivan, "The Pain Catastrophizing Scale: Development and Validation," *Psychological Assessment* 7, no. 4 (1995): 524–532, https://doi.org/10.1037/1040-3590.7.4.524.

20. B. D. Darnall and L. Colloca, "Optimizing Placebo and Minimizing Nocebo to Reduce Pain Catastrophizing, and Opioid Use: A Review of the Science and an Evidence-Informed Clinical Toolkit," *International Review of Neurobiology* 139 (2018): 129–157, https://doi.org/10.1016/bs.irn.2018.07.022.

21. U. Bingel et al., "The Effect of Treatment Expectation on Drug Efficacy: Imaging the Analgesic Benefit of the Opioid Remifentanil," *Science Translation Medicine* 3, no. 70 (2011): https://doi.org/10.1126/scitranslmed.3001244.

22. A. M. Mickle et al., "Relationships Between Pain, Life Stress, Sociodemographics, and Cortisol: Contributions of Pain Intensity and Financial Satisfaction," *Chronic Stress* 4 (2020): 1–12, https://doi.org/10.1177/2470547020975758.

23. D. Y. Lee et al., "Technical and Clinical Aspects of Cortisol as a Biochemical Marker of Chronic Stress," *BMB Reports* 48, no. 5 (2015): 209–216, https:// doi.org/10.5483/bmbrep.2015.48.4.275.

24. J. Basten-Gunther et al., "Optimism and the Experience of Pain: A Systematic Review," *Behavioral Medicine* 45, no. 4 (2019): 323–339, https://doi.org /10.1080/08964289.2018.1517242.

25. K. E. Hannibal and M. D. Bishop, "Chronic Stress, Cortisol Dysfunction, and Pain: A Psychoneuroendocrine Rationale for Stress Management in Pain Rehabilitation," *Physical Therapy* 94 (2014): 1816–1825, https://doi.org /10.2522/ptj.20130597.

26. R. Klinger et al., "Nocebo Effects in Clinical Studies: Hints for Pain Therapy," *Pain Reports* 2, no. 2 (2017): https://doi.org/10.1097/PR9.00000000 00000586.

27. A. N. Gearhardt and E. M. Schulte, "Is Food Addictive? A Review of the Science," *Annual Review of Nutrition* 41 (2021): 387–410, https://doi.org/10.1146 /annurev-nutr-110420-111710.

CHAPTER FOUR: CONSIDER EXERCISE
YOUR FRIEND, NOT YOUR ENEMY

1. E. R. Weibel, C. R. Taylor, and H. Hoppeler, "The Concept of Symmorphosis: A Testable Hypothesis of Structure-Function Relationship," *Proceedings of the National Academy of Sciences* 88, no. 22 (November 1991): https://doi.org/10.1073/pnas.88.22.10357.

2. W. M. Bortz, "A Conceptual Framework of Frailty: A Review," *The Journals of Gerontology Series A: Biological Sciences and Medical Sciences* 57, no. 5 (May 2002): https://doi.org/10.1093/gerona/57.5.m283.

3. Jian Li and Johannes Siegrist, "Physical Activity and Risk of Cardiovascular Disease—A Meta-Analysis of Prospective Cohort Studies," *International Journal of Environmental Research and Public Health* 9, no. 2 (February 2012): 391–407, https://doi.org/10.3390/ijerph9020391.

4. "Prevent Type 2 Diabetes: Talking to Your Patients About Lifestyle Change," *Centers for Disease Control and Prevention*, last modified August 11, 2022, https://www.cdc.gov/diabetes/library/socialmedia/infographics/prevent.html.

5. "Benefits of Exercise for Osteoarthritis," Arthritis Foundation, accessed November 2023; https://www.arthritis.org/health-wellness/healthy-living/physical-activity/getting-started/benefits-of-exercise-for-osteoarthritis; David J. Hunter and Felix Eckstein, "Exercise and Osteoarthritis," *Journal of Anatomy* 214, no. 2 (February 2009): 197–207, https://doi.org/10.1111/j.1469-7580.2008.01013.

6. "Physical Exercise and Dementia," Alzheimer's Society, 2011, https://www.alzheimers.org.uk/about-dementia/risk-factors-and-prevention/physical-exercise. Based on 11 studies.

7. "Physical Exercise and Dementia."

8. Hope Crystal, "Exercise Linked with Lower Risk of 13 Types of Cancer," National Cancer Institute, last modified May 17, 2016, https://www.cancer.gov/about-cancer/causes-prevention/risk/obesity/physical-activity-fact-sheet; "Exercise Linked with Lower Risk of 13 Types of Cancer," American Cancer Society, https://www.cancer.org/latest-news/exercise-linked-with-lower-risk-of-13-types-of-cancer.html; Zeynep Oruç and Muhammed Ali Kaplan,

"Effect of Exercise on Colorectal Cancer Prevention and Treatment," *World Journal of Gastrointestinal Oncology* 11, no. 5 (May 2019): 348–366, https://doi.org/10.4251/wjgo.v11.i5.348.

9. Michael F. Leitzmann et al., "Physical Activity Recommendations and Decreased Risk of Mortality," *Journal of American Medical Association Internal Medicine* 156, no. 22 (2007): 2453–2460, https://doi.org/10.1001/archinte.167.22.2453.

10. I. J. Wallace et al., "Knee Osteoarthritis Has Doubled in Prevalence Since the Mid-20th Century," *Proceedings of the National Academy of Sciences of the United States of America* 114, no. 35 (August 2017): 9332–9336, https://doi.org/10.1073/pnas.1703856114.

11. B. Vanwanseele et al., "Knee Cartilage of Spinal Cord–Injured Patients Displays Progressive Thinning in the Absence of Normal Joint Loading and Movement," *Arthritis & Rheumatism* 46, no. 8 (August 2002): 2073–2078, https://doi.org/10.1002/art.10462.

12. T. L. Racunica, A. J. Teichtahl, Y. Wang, A. E. Wluka, D. R. English, G. G. Giles, R. O'Sullivan, and F. M. Cicuttini, "Effect of Physical Activity on Articular Knee Joint Structures in Community-Based Adults," *Arthritis & Rheumatism* 57, no. 7 (October 2007): 1261–1268, https://doi.org/10.1002/art.22990.

13. F. Berenbaum, I. J. Wallace, D. E. Lieberman, and D. T. Felson, "Modern-Day Environmental Factors in the Pathogenesis of Osteoarthritis," *National Review of Rheumatology* 14, no. 11 (November 2018): 674–681, https://doi.org/10.1038/s41584-018-0073-x.

14. R. F. McLain, "The Nature of Joint Disease in Early Man," *The Iowa Orthopaedic Journal* 11 (1991): 94; C. N. Shaw and J. T. Stock, "Extreme Mobility in the Late Pleistocene? Comparing Limb Biomechanics Among Fossil Homo, Varsity Athletes and Holocene Foragers," *Journal of Human Evolution* 64, no. 4 (April 2013): 242–249, https://doi.org/10.1016/j.jhevol.2013.01.004.

15. A. C. Gelber, M. C. Hochberg, L. A. Mead, N. Y. Wang, F. M. Wigley, and M. J. Klag, "Body Mass Index in Young Men and the Risk of Subsequent Knee and Hip Osteoarthritis," *The American Journal of Medicine* 107, no. 6 (December 1999): 542–548, https://doi.org/10.1016/s0002-9343(99)00292-2.

16. E. M. Roos and N. K. Arden, "Strategies for the Prevention of Knee Osteoarthritis," *Nature Reviews Rheumatology* 12, no. 2 (February 2016): 92–101, https://doi.org/10.1038/nrrheum.2015.135.

17. Edward R. Laskowski, "What Are the Risks of Sitting Too Much?" *Mayo Clinic*, last modified July 13, 2022, https://www.mayoclinic.org/healthy-lifestyle/adult-health/expert-answers/sitting/faq-20058005.

18. A. S. Gersing, B. J. Schwaiger, M. C. Nevitt, G. B. Joseph, N. Chanchek, J. B. Guimaraes, W. J. Mbapte, L. Facchetti, and T. M. Link, "Is Weight Loss Associated with Less Progression of Changes in Knee Articular Cartilage Among Obese and Overweight Patients as Assessed with MR Imaging Over 48 Months? Data from the Osteoarthritis Initiative," *Radiology* 284, no. 2 (August 2017): 508–520, https://doi.org/10.1148/radiol.2017161005.

19. Nina Jullum Kise et al., "Exercise Therapy Versus Arthroscopic Partial Meniscectomy for Degenerative Meniscal Tear in Middle-Aged Patients: Randomized Controlled Trial with Two-Year Follow-up," *British Journal of Sports Medicine* 50 (2016): 1473–1480, https://doi.org/10.1136/bjsports-2016-1374rep.

20. B. J. Shad, G. Wallis, L. J. Van Loon, and J. L. Thompson, "Exercise Prescription for the Older Population: The Interactions Between Physical Activity, Sedentary Time, and Adequate Nutrition in Maintaining Musculoskeletal Health," *Maturitas* 93 (November 2016): 78–82, https://doi.org/10.1016/j.maturitas.2016.05.016.

21. H. Larkin, "Both High- and Low-Dose Exercise Therapy Help Knee Osteoarthritis," *JAMA* 329, no. 7 (2023): 532, https://doi.org/10.1001/jama.2023.0746.

22. Archana Singh-Manoux et al., "Effects of Physical Activity on Cognitive Functioning in Middle Age: Evidence from the Whitehall II Prospective Cohort Study," *American Journal of Public Health* 95 (2005): 2252-2258, https://doi.org/10.2105/AJPH.2004.055574; S. López-Ortiz et al., "Effects of Physical Activity and Exercise Interventions on Alzheimer's Disease: An Umbrella Review of Existing Meta-Analyses," *Journal of Neurology* 270 (2023): 711–725, https://doi.org/10.1007/s00415-022-11454-8.

23. "Brain Basics: The Life and Death of a Neuron," *National Institute of Neurological Disorders and Stroke*, last modified on March 24, 2023, https://

www.ninds.nih.gov/health-information/public-education/brain-basics/brain-basics-life-and-death-neuron.

24. T. Xiao et al., "Association of Bone Mineral Density and Dementia: The Rotterdam Study," *Neurology* (2023): https://doi.org/10.1212/wnl.0000000000207220.

25. K. I. Erickson et al., "Exercise Training Increases Size of Hippocampus and Improves Memory," *Proceedings of the National Academy of Sciences of the United States of America* 108, no. 7 (February 2011): 3017–3022, https://doi.org/10.1073/pnas.1015950108; K. A. Wilckens et al., "Exercise Interventions Preserve Hippocampal Volume: A Meta-Analysis," *Hippocampus* 31, no. 3 (March 2021): 335–347, https://doi.org/10.1002/hipo.23292; K. I. Erickson, D. L. Miller, and K. A. Roecklein, "The Aging Hippocampus: Interactions Between Exercise, Depression, and BDNF," *Neuroscientist* 18, no. 1 (February 2012): 82–97, https://doi.org/10.1177/1073858410397054.

26. C. W. Cotman and N. C. Berchtold, "Exercise: A Behavioral Intervention to Enhance Brain Health and Plasticity," *Trends in Neurosciences* 25, no. 6 (June 2002): 295–301, https://doi.org/10.1016/s0166-2236(02)02143-4; R. Bonanni et al., "Physical Exercise and Health: A Focus on Its Protective Role in Neurodegenerative Diseases," *Journal of Functional Morphology and Kinesiology* 7, no. 2 (April 2022): 38, https://doi.org/10.3390/jfmk7020038.

27. K. I. Erickson, A. G. Gildengers, and M. A. Butters, "Physical Activity and Brain Plasticity in Late Adulthood," *Dialogues in Clinical Neuroscience* (April 2022): 99–108, https://doi.org/10.31887/DCNS.2013.15.1/kerickson.

28. T. F. Yuan, F. Paes, O. Arias-Carrión, N. Barbosa Ferreira Rocha, A. Souza de Sá Filho, and S. Machado, "Neural Mechanisms of Exercise: Anti-Depression, Neurogenesis, and Serotonin Signaling," *CNS & Neurological Disorders-Drug Targets* (formerly *Current Drug Targets-CNS & Neurological Disorders*) 14, no. 10 (December 2015): 1307–1311, https://doi.org/10.2174/1871527315666151111124402.

29. S. Heijnen, B. Hommel, A. Kibele, and L. S. Colzato, "Neuromodulation of Aerobic Exercise—A Review," *Frontiers in Psychology* 6, no. 1890 (January 2016): https://doi.org/10.3389/fpsyg.2015.01890.

30. S. N. Young, "How to Increase Serotonin in the Human Brain Without Drugs," *Journal of Psychiatry & Neuroscience* 32, no. 6 (November 2007):

394–399; M. O. Melancon, D. Lorrain, and I. J. Dionne, "Exercise and Sleep in Aging: Emphasis on Serotonin," *Pathologie-Biologie* 62, no. 5 (October 2014): 276–283, https://doi.org/10.1016/j.patbio.2014.07.004; Makoto Kondo and Shoichi Shimada, "Serotonin and Exercise-Induced Brain Plasticity," *Neurotransmitter* 2, no. e793 (2015): 10-14800; T. F. Yuan et al., "Neural Mechanisms of Exercise: Anti-Depression, Neurogenesis, and Serotonin Signaling," *CNS & Neurological Disorders-Drug Targets* (formerly *Current Drug Targets-CNS & Neurological Disorders*) 14, no. 10 (December 2015): 1307–1311, https://doi.org/10.2174/1871527315666151111124402.

31. Susan A. Carlson et al., "Percentage of Deaths Associated with Inadequate Physical Activity in the United States," *Preventing Chronic Disease: Public Health Research, Practice, and Policy* 15, no. 170354 (2018): http://dx.doi.org/10.5888/pcd18.170354.

32. E. Roddy, W. Zhang, and M. Doherty, "Aerobic Walking or Strengthening Exercise for Osteoarthritis of the Knee? A Systematic Review," *Annals of the Rheumatic Diseases* 64, no. 4 (April 2005): 544–548, https://doi.org/10.1136/ard.2004.028746; L. Brosseau et al., "Efficacy of Aerobic Exercises for Osteoarthritis (Part II): A Meta-Analysis," *Physical Therapy Reviews* 9, no. 3 (September 2004): 125–145; J. Brosseau et al., "The Ottawa Panel Clinical Practice Guidelines for the Management of Knee Osteoarthritis. Part Three: Aerobic Exercise Programs," *Clinical Rehabilitation* 31, no. 5 (May 2017): 612–624, https://doi.org/10.1177/0269215517691085.

33. C. Juhl et al., "Impact of Exercise Type and Dose on Pain and Disability in Knee Osteoarthritis: A Systematic Review and Meta-Regression Analysis of Randomized Controlled Trials," *Arthritis & Rheumatology* 66, no. 3 (March 2014): 622–636, https://doi.org/10.1002/art.38290; S. L. Goh et al., "Relative Efficacy of Different Exercises for Pain, Function, Performance and Quality of Life in Knee and Hip Osteoarthritis: Systematic Review and Network Meta-Analysis," *Sports Medicine* 49 (May 2019): 743–761, https://doi.org/10.1007/s40279-019-01082-0; M. Henriksen et al., "Comparable Effects of Exercise and Analgesics for Pain Secondary to Knee Osteoarthritis: A Meta-Analysis of Trials Included in Cochrane Systematic Reviews," *Journal of Comparative Effectiveness Research* 5, no. 4 (July 2016): 417–431, https://doi.org/10.2217/cer-2016-0007; J. M. Gwinnutt et al., "2021 EULAR

Recommendations Regarding Lifestyle Behaviours and Work Participation to Prevent Progression of Rheumatic and Musculoskeletal Diseases," *Annals of the Rheumatic Diseases* 82, no. 1 (January 2023): 48–56, https://doi.org /10.1136/annrheumdis-2021-222020.

34. Matthew M. Robinson et al., "Enhanced Protein Translation Underlines Improved Metabolic and Physical Adaptations to Different Exercise Training Modes in Young and Old Humans," *Cell Metabolism* 22 (March 2017): 581–592, http://dx.doi.org/10.1016/j.cmet.2017.02.009; I. Lozano-Montoya et al., "Nonpharmacological Iterventions to Treat Physical Frailty and Sarcopenia in Older Patients: A Systematic Overview–the SENATOR Project ONTOP Series," *Clinical Interventions in Aging* (April 2017): 721–740, https://doi.org/10.2147/CIA.S132496; D. Beckwée et al., "Sarcopenia Guidelines Development Group of the Belgian Society of Gerontology and Geriatrics (BSGG). Exercise Interventions for the Prevention and Treatment of Sarcopenia. A Systematic Umbrella Review," *Journal of Nutrition, Health & Aging* 23 (June 2019): 494–502, https://doi.org/10.1007/s12603-019-1196-8.

35. D. Tarantino et al., "High-Intensity Training for Knee Osteoarthritis: A Narrative Review," *Sports* 11, no. 4 (April 2023): 91, https://doi.org/10.3390 /sports11040091.

36. A. J. Cruz-Jentoft and A. A. Sayer, "Sarcopenia," *Lancet* 393, no. 10191 (June 2019): 2636–2346, https://doi.org/10.1016/S0140-6736(19)31138-9.

37. H. B. Bårdstu et al., "Effectiveness of a Resistance Training Program on Physical Function, Muscle Strength, and Body Composition in Community-Dwelling Older Adults Receiving Home Care: A Cluster-Randomized Controlled Trial," *European Review of Aging and Physical Activity* 17, no. 1 (December 2020): 11, https://doi.org/10.1186/s11556-020-00243-9; J. M. Dickinson, E. Volpi, and B. B. Rasmussen, "Exercise and Nutrition to Target Protein Synthesis Impairments in Aging Skeletal Muscle," *Exercise and Sport Sciences Reviews* 41, no. 4 (October 2013): 216, https://doi.org/10.1097 /JES.0b013e3182a4e699; M. Tieland et al., "Protein Supplementation Increases Muscle Mass Gain During Prolonged Resistance-Type Exercise Training in Frail Elderly People: A Randomized, Double-Blind, Placebo-Controlled Trial," *Journal of the American Medical Directors Association* 13, no. 8 (October 2012): 713–719, https://doi.org/10.1016/j.jamda.2012.05.020.

38. R. C. Cassilhas et al., "The Impact of Resistance Exercise on the Cognitive Function of the Elderly," *Medicine & Science in Sports & Exercise* 39, no. 8 (August 2007): 1401–1407, https://doi.org/10.1249/mss.0b013e318060111f; J. M. del Campo Cervantes, M. H. Macías Cervantes, and R. Monroy Torres, "Effect of a Resistance Training Program on Sarcopenia and Functionality of the Older Adults Living in a Nursing Home," *Journal of Nutrition Health & Aging* 23 (November 2019): 829–836, https://doi.org/10.1007/s12603-019-1261-3.

39. B. J. Schoenfeld et al., "Longer Interset Rest Periods Enhance Muscle Strength and Hypertrophy in Resistance-Trained Men," *Journal of Strength and Conditioning Research* 30, no. 7 (July 2016): 1805–1812, https://doi.org/10.1519/JSC.0000000000001272.

40. A. J. Cruz-Jentoft et al., "Nutritional Strategies for Maintaining Muscle Mass and Strength from Middle Age to Later Life: A Narrative Review," *Maturitas* 132 (February 2020): 57–64, https://doi.org/10.1016/j.maturitas.2019.11.007.

41. D. Eglseer et al., "Nutritional and Exercise Interventions in Individuals with Sarcopenic Obesity Around Retirement Age: A Systematic Review and Meta-Analysis," *Nutrition Reviews* 81, no. 9 (March 2023): 1077-1090, https://doi.org/10.1093/nutrit/nuad007.

42. A. C. Cunha et al., "Effect of Global Posture Reeducation and of Static Stretching on Pain, Range of Motion, and Quality of Life in Women with Chronic Neck Pain: A Randomized Clinical Trial," *Clinics* 63, no. 6 (2008): 763–770, https://doi.org/10.1590/s1807-59322008000600010; A. F. Carvalho et al., "Effects of Lumbar Stabilization and Muscular Stretching on Pain, Disabilities, Postural Control and Muscle Activation in Pregnant Woman with Low Back Pain," *European Journal of Physical and Rehabilitation Medicine* 56, no. 3 (January 2020): 297–306, https://doi.org/10.23736/S1973-9087.20.06086-4.

CHAPTER FIVE: OPTIMIZE WITH DIET

1. "How We Poison Our Children" (PDF), *New York Times*, May 13, 1858.

2. Cristin E. Kearns, Laura A. Schmidt, and Stanton A. Glantz, "Sugar Industry and Coronary Heart Disease Research." *JAMA International*

Medicine 176, no. 11 (November 2016): 1680–1685, https://doi.org/10.1001/jamainternmed.2016.5394.

3. Samir Faruque et al., "The Dose Makes the Poison: Sugar and Obesity in the United States—A Review," *Polish Journal of Food and Nutrition Sciences* 69, no. 3 (2019): 219–233, https://doi.org/10.31883/pjfns/110735.

4. C. A. Monteiro et al., "The Food System. Ultra-Processing: The Big Issue for Nutrition, Disease, Health, Well-Being. [Commentary]." *World Nutrition* 3, no. 12 (December 2012): 527–569.

5. M. J. Gibney, "Ultraprocessed Foods and Their Application to Nutrition Policy," *Nutrition Today* 55, no. 1 (2020): 16–21, https://doi.org/10.1097/NT.0000000000000393.

6. Andrea K. Garber and Robert H. Lustig, "Is Fast Food Addictive?" *Journal of Current Drug Abuse Reviews* 4, no. 3 (September 2011): 146–162, https://doi.org/10.2174/1874473711104030146.

7. Barbara J. Rolls et al., "Properties of Ultra Processed Foods That Can Drive Excess Intake," *Nutrition Today* 55, no. 3 (May 2020): https://doi.org/10.1097/NT.0000000000000410.

8. M. M. Lane et al., "Ultraprocessed Food and Chronic Noncommunicable Diseases: A Systematic Review and Meta-Analysis of 43 Observational Studies," *Obesity Reviews* 22, no. 3 (2021): 1–19, https://doi.org/10.1111/obr.13146.

9. L. Li et al., "Selected Nutrient Analyses of Fresh, Fresh-Stored, and Frozen Fruits and Vegetables," *Journal of Food Composition and Analysis* 59 (2017): 8–17, https://doi.org/10.1016/j.jfca.2017.02.002.

10. Kerstin N. Vokinger et al., "Therapeutic Value of Drugs Granted Accelerated Approval or Conditional Marketing Authorization in the US and Europe from 2007 to 2021," *JAMA Health Forum* 3, no. 8 (2022): https://doi.org/10.1001/jamahealthforum.2022.2685.

11. A. B. Keys, *Seven Countries: A Multivariate Analysis of Death and Coronary Heart Disease* (Cambridge, MA: Harvard University Press, 1980).

12. W. C. Willet et al., "Mediterranean Diet Pyramid: A Cultural Model for Healthy Eating," *American Journal of Clinical Nutrition* 61, no. 6 (1995):1402S-1406S, https://doi.org/10.1093/ajcn/61.6.1402S.

13. Willet et al., "Mediterranean Diet Pyramid."

14. M. Finicelli et al., "The Mediterranean Diet: An Update of the Clinical Trials," *Nutrients* 14, no. 2956 (2022): https://doi.org/10.3390/nu14142956.

15. Robert P. Heaney, "Making Sense of the Science of Sodium," *Nutrition Today* 50, no. 2 (March 2015): 63–68, https://doi.org/10.1097/NT.0000000000000084.

16. Aseem Malhotra, *A Statin-Free Life* (Hodder & Stoughton/Hachette UK, 2021), 132.

17. Alice H. Lichtenstein, "Dietary Sodium: Let's Focus on What We Know and How to Move Forward," *Nutrition Today* 54, no. 6 (November 2019): https://doi.org/10.1097/01.NT.0000604480.64658.44.

18. Mehmet C. Oz and Michael F. Roizen, *You: The Owner's Manual: An Insider's Guide to the Body That Will Make You Healthier and Stronger* (New York: William Morrow, 2013), 501.

19. Ekpor Anyimah-Ackah et al., "Exposures and risks of arsenic, cadmium, lead, and mercury in cocoa beans and cocoa-based foods: a systematic review," *Food Quality and Safety* 3, no. 1 (2019): 1–8; Supriya Joshi, "Potential risks of cadmium toxicity from cocoa based products: a review," *International Journal of Current Medical and Pharmaceutical Research* 7 (2021): 5650–5653.

20. M. Flores-Valdez et al., "Identification and Quantification of Adulterants in Coffee (*Coffea arabica L.*) Using FT-MIR Spectroscopy Couple with Chemometrics," *Foods* 9, no. 7 (2020): 851, https://doi.org/10.3390/foods9070851.

21. GBD 2016 Alcohol Collaborators, "Alcohol Use and Burden for 195 Countries and Territories, 1990–2016: A Systematic Analysis for the Global Burden of Disease Study 2016," *Lancet* 392, no. 10152 (2018): 1015–1035, https://doi.org/10.1016/S0140-6736(18)31310-2.

22. Angela M. Malek et al., "Dietary Sources of Sugars and Calories," *Nutrition Today*, 54, no. 6, (November 2019): 296–303, https://doi.org/10.1097/NT.0000000000000378.

23. Jotham Suez et al., "Artificial Sweeteners Induce Glucose Intolerance by Altering the Gut Microbiota," *Nature* 514 (2014): 181–186, https://doi.org/10.1038/Nature13793.

24. Densie Webb, "Pasta's History and Role in Healthful Diets,"*Nutrition Today*54, no. 5, (September 2019). https://doi.org/10.1097/NT.0000000000000364.

25. B. H. Arjmandi et al., "Soy Protein May Alleviate Osteoarthritis Symptoms," *Phyto-Med* 11, no. 7–8 (2004): 567–75, https://doi.org10.1016/j.phymed.2003.11.001.

26. F. Oliviero et al., "How the Mediterranean Diet and Some of Its Components Modulate Inflammatory Pathways in Arthritis," *Swiss Medical Weekly* 145, no. 14190 (2015): https://doi.org/10.4414/smw.2015.14190.

27. M. D. Kontogianni et al., "Adherence to the Mediterranean Diet and Serum Uric Acid: The ATTICA Study," *Scandinavian Journal of Rheumatology* 41 (2012): 442–449, https://doi.org/10.3109/03009 742.2012.679964.

28. G. Musumeci et al., "Extra-Virgin Olive Oil Diet and Mild Physical Activity Prevent Cartilage Degeneration in an Osteoarthritis Model: An In Vivo and In Vitro Study on Lubricin Expression," *Journal of Nutritional Biochemistry* 24, no. 12 (December 2013): 2064–2075, https://doi.org/10.1016/j.jnutbio.2013.07.007. PMID: 24369033.

29. I. Morales-Ivorra et al., "Osteoarthritis and the Mediterranean Diet: A Systematic Review," *Nutrients* 10, no. 8 (August 2018): 1030, https://doi.org/10.3390/nu10081030. PMID: 30087302.

30. B. Harrison and D. Symmons, "Early Inflammatory Polyarthritis: Results from the Norfolk Arthritis Register with a Review of the Literature. II. Outcome at Three Years," *Rheumatology* 39, no. 9 (September 2000): 939–949, https://doi.org/10.1093/rheumatology/39.9.939.

31. N. Veronese et al., "Mediterranean Diet and Knee Osteoarthritis Outcomes: A Longitudinal Cohort Study," *Clinical Nutrition* 38, no. 6 (December 2019): 2735–2739, https://doi.org/10.1016/j.clnu.2018.11.032.

32. A. Sadeghi et al., "Effects of a Mediterranean Diet Compared with the Low-Fat Diet on Patients with Knee Osteoarthritis: A Randomized Feeding Trial." *International Journal of Clinical Practice* 7275192 (January 2022): https://doi.org/10.1155/2022/7275192.

33. C. Tsigalou et al., "Mediterranean Diet as a Tool to Combat Inflammation and Chronic Diseases: An Overview," *Biomedicines* 8, no. 7 (July 2020): 201, https://doi.org/10.3390/biomedicines8070201.

34. H. S. Han et al., "Erratum to: Relationship Between Total Fruit and Vegetable Intake and Self-Reported Knee Pain in Older Adults," *Journal of Nutritional Health Aging* 26, no. 904 (2022): https://doi.org/10.1007/s12603-021-1602–x.

35. A. E. Connelly et al., "Modifiable Lifestyle Factors Are Associated with Lower Pain Levels in Adults with Knee Osteoarthritis," *Pain Research and Management* 20, no. 5 (September 2015): 241–248, https://doi.org/10.1155/2015/389084.

36. M. Hatori et al., "Time-Restricted Feeding Without Reducing Caloric Intake Prevents Metabolic Diseases in Mice Fed a High-Fat Diet," *Cell Metabolism* 15, no. 6 (June 2012) 848–860, https://doi.org/10.1016/j.cmet.2012.04.019.

37. Katelyn M. Mellion and Grandon T. Grover, "Obesity, Bariatric Surgery, and Hip/Knee Arthroplasty Outcomes," *Surgery Clinics of North America* 101 (2021): 295–305, https://doi.org/1-.1016/j.suc.2020.12.011.

38. P. J. Belmont et al., "Thirty-Day Postoperative Complications and Mortality Following Total Knee Arthroplasty: Incidence and Risk Factors Among a National Sample of 15,321 Patients," *Journal of Bone & Joint Surgery America* 96, no. 1 (2014): 20–6, https://doi.org/10.2106/JBJS.M.00018; T. K. Fehring et al., "The Obesity Epidemic: Its Effect on Total Joint Arthroplasty," *Journal of Arthroplasty* 22, no. 6 (2007): 71–76, https://doi.org/10.1016/j.arth.2007.04.014; H. M. Kremers et al., "The Effect of Obesity on Direct Medical Costs in Total Knee Arthroplasty," *Journal of Bone and Joint Surgery* 96, no. 9 (2014): 718–724, https://doi.org/10.2106/JBJS.N.00019.

39. Christopher Edwards et al., "The Effects of Bariatric Surgery Weight Loss on Knee Pain in Patients with Osteoarthritis of the Knee," *Arthritis* no. 504189 (2012): https://doi.org/10.1155/2012/504189.

40. J. M. Hootman et al., "Updated Projected Prevalence of Self-Reported Doctor Diagnosed Arthritis and Arthritis-Attributable Activity Limitation Among US Adults, 2015–2040," *Arthritis & Rheumatology* 68, no. 7 (2016): 1582–1587, https://doi.org/10.1002/art.39692.

41. Tony Robbins, *Life Force* (New York: Simon & Schuster, 2022), 496.

42. Greta M. Massetti et al. "Excessive Weight Gain, Obesity, and Cancer," *JAMA* 318, no. 20 (November 2017): 1975–1976, https://doi.org/10.1001/jama.2017.15519; "Health Impacts of Obesity: An Overview," *Obesity Evidence Hub*, accessed November 2023, https://www.obesityevidencehub.org.au/collections/impacts/health-impacts-of-obesity.

43. Edwards et al., "The Effects of Bariatric Surgery Weight Loss on Knee Pain in Patients with Osteoarthritis of the Knee."

44. Amir Zarrinpar et al., "Diet and Feeding Pattern Affect the Diurnal Dynam-
    ics of the Gut Microbiome," *Journal of Cell Metabolism* 20 (December 2014):
    1006–1017, https://doi.org/ 10.1016/j.cmet.2014.11.008; B. H. Goodpaster et
    al., "Skeletal Muscle Lipid Accumulation in Obesity, Insulin Resistance, and
    Type 2 Diabetes," *Pediatric Diabetes* 5 (2004): 219–226.

45. Alice A. Gibson, and Amanda Swainsbury, "Strategies to Improve Adherence
    to Dietary Weight Loss Interventions in Research and Real-World Settings,"
    Behavioral Science 7, no. 4 (2017): https://doi.org/10.3390/bs7030044.

46. Mark P. Mattson et al., "Meal Frequency and Timing in Health and Disease," *Pro-
    ceedings of the National Academy of Sciences of the United States of America* 111, no.
    47 (November 2014): 16647–16653. https://doi.org/10.1073/pnas.1413965111.

47. Gurinder Bains et al., "Four Weeks of 16:8 Time-Restricted Feeding on
    Stress, Sleep, Quality of Life, Hunger Level, and Body Composition in
    Healthy Adults: A Pilot Study on Wellness Optimization," *Journal of Wellness*
    (November 2021): https://doi.org/10.18297/jwellness/vol3/iss2/10.

48. M. P. Mattson, V. D. Longo, and M. Harvie, "Impact of Intermittent Fast-
    ing on Health and Disease Processes," *Ageing Research Reviews* 39 (October
    2017): 46–58, https://doi.org/10.1016/j.arr.2016.10.005.

49. Robbins, *Life Force*, 289.

50. A. J. Carlson and F. R. Hoelzel, "Apparent Prolongation of the Life Span
    of Rats by Intermittent Fasting: One Figure," *Journal of Nutrition* 31, no. 3
    (March 1946): 363–375, https://doi.org/10.1093/jn/31.3.363; David A. Sin-
    clair, *Lifespan: Why We Age and Why We Don't Have To* (New York: Simon
    and Schuster, 2019), 95–96.

51. Amy Locke et al., "Diets for Health: Goals and Guidelines," *American Acad-
    emy of Family Physicians* 97, no. 11 (2018): 721–728.

CHAPTER SIX: SLEEP MATTERS MIGHTILY

1. Matthew Walker, *Why We Sleep* (New York: Simon and Schuster, 2017), 145.

2. Walker, *Why We Sleep*, 136.

3. Walker, *Why We Sleep*, 136.

4. Some researchers discuss a fourth NREM sleep stage that is slightly deeper
   than N3, but most still discuss three non-REM stages.

5. M. Wittman et al., "Social Jetlag: Misalignment of Biological and Social Time," *Chronobiology International* 23, no. 1–2 (2006): 497–509, https://doi.org/10.1080/07420520500545979.

6. Ravi Allada and Joseph Bass, "Circadian Mechanisms in Medicine," *New England Journal of Medicine* 384, no. 6 (2021): 550–561, https://doi.org/10.1056/NEJMra1802337.

7. Deanna Marie Arble et al., "Circadian Disruption and Metabolic Disease: Findings from Animal Models," *Best Practices and Research in Clinical Endocrinology and Metabolism* 24, no. 5 (October 2010): 785–800, https://doi.org/0.106/j.beem.2010.08.003; Frank A. J. L. Scheer et al., "Adverse Metabolic and Cardiovascular Consequences of Circadian Misalignment," *Proceedings of the National Academy of Sciences* 106, no. 11 (March 2009): 4453–4458. https://doi.org/10.1073/pnas.0808180106; Kenneth Wright et al., "Influence of Sleep Deprivation and Circadian Misalignment on Cortisol, Inflammatory Markers, and Cytokine Balance," *Brain Behavior Immunity* 47 (July 2015): 24–34, https://doi.org/10.1016/j.bbi.2015.01.004; Kelly G. Baron et al., "Role of Sleep Timing in Caloric Intake and BMI," *Obesity* 19 (2011): 1374–1381, https://doi.org/10.1038/oby.2011.100; Josiane L. Broussard et al., "Disturbances of Sleep and Circadian Rhythms: Novel Risks Factors for Obesity," *Current Opinion in Endocrinology, Diabetes, and Obesity* 23, no. 5 (October 2016): 353–359, https://doi.org/10.1097/MED; Gregory D. M. Potter et al., "Circadian Rhythm and Sleep Disruption: Causes, Metabolic Consequences, and Countermeasures," *Endocrine Reviews* 37, no. 6 (December 2016): 584–608, https://doi.org/10.1210/er.2016-1083.

8. Satchin Panda, *The Circadian Code: Lose Weight, Supercharge Your Energy, and Transform Your Health from Morning to Midnight* (New York: Rodale, 2018).

9. Hatori et al., "Time-Restricted Feeding Without Reducing Caloric Intake Prevents Metabolic Diseases in Mice Fed a High-Fat Diet."

10. Ali Mobasheri and Mark Batt, "An Update on the Pathophysiology of Osteoarthritis," *Annals of Physical and Rehabilitation Medicine* 59, no. 5-6 (2016): 333-339.

11. Shu-qun Shi et al., "Circadian Disruption Leads to Insulin Resistance and Obesity," *Current Biology* 23, no. 5 (2013): 372–381.

CHAPTER SEVEN: SUPPLEMENTS THAT OFFER SUPPORT

1. Bashar Saad, Hassan Azaizeh, and Omar Said, "Tradition and Perspectives of Arab Herbal Medicine: A Review," *Evidence-Based Complementary and Alternative Medicine* 2, no. 4 (2005): 475–479, https://doi.org/10.1093/ecam/neh133.

2. Louis E. Grivetti, "Herbs, Spices, and Flavoring Agents: Part 1: Old World Contributions," *Nutrition Today* 51, no. 3 (May 2016): https://doi.org//1097/NT.0000000000000149; Louis E. Grivetti, "Herbs, Spices, and Flavoring Agents: Part 2: New World Contributions," *Nutrition Today*, 51, no. 5, (September 2016): https://doi.org/10/1097/NT.0000000000000171; Louis E. Grivetti, "Herbs, Spices, and Flavoring Agents: Part 3: The Fusion—Development of New Cuisines (Early Exploration Accounts and Information From Early Settlements in Virginia and New England," *Nutrition Today* 51, no. 4 (July 2016): https://doi.org/10/1097/NT.0000000000000166; Louis E. Grivetti, "Herbs, Spices, and Flavoring Agents: Part 4: The Fusion—The Development of New Cuisines During the Colonial, Revolutionary, and Federal Periods," *Nutrition Today* 51, no. 6 (November 2016): https://doi.org/10/1097/NT.0000000000000181; Louis E. Grivetti, "Herbs, Spices, and Flavoring Agents: Part 5: Fusion of Herbs and Spices in the 19th-Century and Into the 21st Century North American Culture," *Nutrition Today* 52, no. 1 (January 2017): https://doi.org/10/1097/NT.0000000000000189.

3. Jeff Moore, Amanda McClain, and Mee Young Hong, "Dietary Supplement Use in the United States: Prevalence, Trends, Pros, and Cons," *Nutrition Today* 55, no. 4 (July 2020): https://doi.org/ 10.1097/NT.0000000000000402.

4. Paul Gougis et al., "Potential Cytochrome P450–Mediated Pharmacokinetic Interactions Between Herbs, Food, and Dietary Supplements and Cancer Treatments," *Critical Review in Oncology/Hematology* (2021): 103342, https://doi.org/10.1016/jcritrevonc.2021.103342; Vanny Sharma et al., "Pharmacodynamic and Pharmacokinetic Interactions of Herbs with Prescribed Drugs: A Review," *Plant Archives* 21, no. 1 (2021): 185–198, https://doi.org/ 10.51470/PLANTARCHIVES.2021.v21.S1.033.

CHAPTER EIGHT: THERAPIES AND ALTERNATIVE NATURAL TREATMENTS

1. Kevin Cheng et al., "Mechanisms and Pathways of Pain Photobiomodulation: A Narrative Review," *Journal of Pain* 22, no. 7 (2021): 763–777, https://doi.org/10.1016/j.jpain.2021.02.005; Mohab M. Ibrahim et al., "Long-Lasting Antinociceptive Effects of Green Light in Acute and Chronic Pain in Rats," *Pain* 158, no. 2 (2017): 347–360, https://doi.org/10.1097/j.pain.0000000000000767.

2. Jacob R. Bumgarner, and Randy J. Nelson, "Light at Night and Disrupted Circadian Rhythms Alter Physiology and Behavior," *Integrative and Comparative Biology* 61, no. 3 (2021): 1160–1169, https://doi.org/10.1093/icb/icab017.

3. Yueh-Ling Hsieh et al., "Low-Level Laser Therapy Alleviates Neuropathic Pain and Promotes Function Recovery in Rats with Chronic Constriction Injury: Possible Involvements in Hypoxia-Inducible Factor 1α (HIF-1α)," *Journal of Comparative Neurology* 520, no. 13 (2012): 2903–2916, https://doi.org/10.1002/cne.23072; Rajesh Khanna et al., "Development and Characterization of an Injury-Free Model of Functional Pain in Rats by Exposure to Red Light," *Journal of Pain* 20, no. 11 (2019): 1293–1306, https://doi.org/10.1016/j.jpain.2019.04.008.

4. Hsieh et al., "Low-Level Laser Therapy Alleviates Neuropathic Pain and Promotes Function Recovery in Rats with Chronic Constriction Injury"; Khanna et al., "Development and Characterization of an Injury-Free Model of Functional Pain in Rats by Exposure to Red Light."

5. Mohab M. Ibrahim et al., "Long-Lasting Antinociceptive Effects of Green Light in Acute and Chronic Pain in Rats," *Pain* 158, no. 2 (2017): 347–360, https://doi.org/10.1097/j.pain.0000000000000767.

6. Gustavo Balbinot et al., "Photobiomodulation Therapy Partially Restores Cartilage Integrity and Reduces Chronic Pain Behavior in a Rat Model of Osteoarthritis: Involvement of Spinal Glial Modulation," *Cartilage* 13, no. 2 (2021): 1309S–1321S, https://doi.org/10.1177/1947603519876338; Helen J.

Burgess et al., "An Open Trial of Morning Bright Light Treatment Among US Military Veterans with Chronic Low Back Pain: A Pilot Study," *Pain Medicine* 20, no. 4 (2019): 770–778, https://doi.org/10.1093/pm/pny174; John W. Burns et al., "Morning Bright Light Treatment for Chronic Low Back Pain: Potential Impact on the Volatility of Pain, Mood, Function, and Sleep," *Pain Medicine* 21, no. 6 (2020): 1153–1161, https://doi.org/10.1093/pm/pnz235; Martin Bjørn Stausholm et al., "Efficacy of Low-Level Laser Therapy on Pain and Disability in Knee Osteoarthritis: Systematic Review and Meta-Analysis of Randomised Placebo-Controlled Trials," *BMJ Open* 9, no. 10 (2019): https://doi.org/10.1136/bmjopen-2019-031142.

7. Stausholm et al., "Efficacy of Low-Level Laser Therapy on Pain and Disability in Knee Osteoarthritis: Systematic Review and Meta-Analysis of Randomised Placebo-Controlled Trials."

8. Jonathan A. Lindquist and Peter R. Mertens, "Cold Shock Proteins: From Cellular Mechanisms to Pathophysiology and Disease," *Cell Communication and Signaling* 16, no. 1 (2018): 1–14, https://doi.org/10.1186/s12964-018-0274-6.

9. Pei-Chi Chou and Heng-Yi Chu, "Clinical Efficacy of Acupuncture on Rheumatoid Arthritis and Associated Mechanisms: A Systemic Review," *Evidence-Based Complementary and Alternative Medicine* 8596918 (2018): https://doi.org/10.1155/2018/8596918.

10. Jorge Vas et al., "Acupuncture as a Complementary Therapy to the Pharmacological Treatment of Osteoarthritis of the Knee: Randomised Controlled Trial," *BMJ* 329, no. 7476 (2004): 1216, https://doi.org/10.1136/bmj.38238.601447.3A.

CHAPTER NINE: CUE UP QUESTIONS TO ASK YOUR DOCTOR

1. Monica Van Such et al., "Extent of Diagnostic Agreement Among Medical Referrals," *Journal of Evaluation in Clinical Practice* 23, no. 4 (August 2017): 870–874, https://doi.org/10.1111/jep.12747.

APPENDIX I: LIST OF SUPPLEMENTS

1. S. Brien et al., "Bromelain as a Treatment for Osteoarthritis: A Review of Clinical Studies," *Evidence Based Complementary and Alternative Medicine* 1, no. 3 (December 2004): 251–257, https://doi.org/10.1093/ecam/neh035.

2. Vipin Arora, James N. Campbell, and Man-Kyo Chung, "Fight Fire with Fire: Neurobiology of Capsaicin-Induced Analgesia for Chronic Pain," *Pharmacology & Therapeutics* 220 (2021): 107743, https://doi.org/10.1016/j .pharmthera.2020.107743.

3. W. Johnson and Junior McRorie, "Evidence-Based Approach to Fiber Supplements and Clinically Meaningful Health Benefits, Part 1: What to Look for and How to Recommend an Effective Fiber Therapy," *Nutrition Today* 50, no. 2 (March 2015): https://doi.org 10.1097/NT.000000000000089; W. Johnson and Junior McRorie, "Evidence-Based Approach to Fiber Supplements and Clinically Meaningful Health Benefits, Part 2: What to Look for and How to Recommend an Effective Fiber Therapy," *Nutrition Today* 50, no. 2, (March 2015): https://doi.org10.1097/NT.000000000000082.

4. M. Tam et al., "Possible Roles of Magnesium on the Immune System," *European Journal of Clinical Nutrition* 57 (2003): 1193–1197, https://doi .org/10.1038/sh.ejcn.1601689.

5. Adela Hruby and Nicola M. McKeown, "Magnesium Deficiency," *Nutrition Today* 51, no. 3 (May 2016): 121–127, https://doi.org10.1097/nt.0000 000000000158.

6. Mario Barbagallo et al., "Magnesium Homeostasis and Aging," *Magnesium Research* 22, no. 4 (2009): 235–246, https://doi.org/10.1684/mrh.2009.0187.

7. S. Emila and S. Swaminathan, "Role of Magnesium in Health and Disease," *Journal of Experimental Sciences* 4, no. 2 (2013): 32–43.

8. Juliana de Aguiar Pastore Silva et al., "Omega-3 Supplements for Patients in Chemotherapy and/or Radiotherapy: A Systematic Review," *Clinical Nutrition* 34 (2015): 359–366, https://doi.org/10.1016/j.clnu.2014.11.005.

9. Shima Jazayeri et al., "Comparison of Therapeutic Effects of Omega-3 Fatty Acid Eicosapentaenoic Acid and Fluoxetine, Separately and in Combination,

in Major Depressive Disorder," *Australian and New Zealand Journal of Psychiatry* 42 (2008): 192–198, https://doi.org/10.1080/00048670701827275.

10. Amy H.R. Wood et al., "Dietary and Supplemental Long-Chain Omega-3 Fatty Acids as Moderators of Cognitive Impairment and Alzheimer's Disease," *European Journal of Nutrition*, 61 (2022): 589–604, https://doi.org/10/1007/x00394-021-02655-4.

11. W. G. Christen et al., "Dietary OB RA and Fish Intake and Incident Age-Related Molecular Degeneration in Women," *Archive of Journal of Ophtalmology* 129 (March 2011): 192–199, https://doi.org/10.1001/archophthalmol.2011.34.

12. Betsy McKay, "New Shot for Fish Oil—Into the Bloodstream," *Wall Street Journal,* September 8, 2022, https://www.wsj.com/articles/a-new-shot-at-using-fish-oil-11662385576.

13. Keith Singletary, "Rosemary: An Overview of Potential Health Benefits," *Nutrition Today* 51, no. 2 (March 2016): https://doi.org/10.1097/NT.0000000000000146.

14. Keith Singletary, "Saffron: Potential Health Benefits," *Nutrition Today* 55, no. 6 (November 2020): https://doi.org/10.1097/NT.000000000000449.

15. Z. Hamidi et al., "The Effect of Saffron Supplement on Clinical Outcomes and Metabolic Profiles in Patients with Active Rheumatoid Arthritis: A Randomized, Double-Blind, Placebo-Controlled Clinical Trial," *Phytotherapy Research* 34 (2020): 1650–1658, https://doi.org/10.1002/ptr.6633.

16. Keith Singletary, "Turmeric: Potential Health Benefits," *Nutrition Today* 55, no. 1 (January 2020): https://doi.org/10.1097/NT.0000000000000392.

17. Inga Wessels et al., "Zinc as a Gatekeeper of Immune Function," *Nutrients* 9, no. 1286 (2017): https://doi.org/10.3390/nu9121286.

18. Ananda S. Prasad et al., "Zinc Supplementation Decreases Incidence of Infections in the Elderly: Effect of Zinc on Generation of Cytokines and Oxidative Stress," *American Journal of Clinical Nutrition* 85 (2007): 837–844, https://doi.org/10.1093/ajcn/85.3.837.

19. Ananda S. Prasad, "Impact of the Discovery of Human Zinc Deficiency on Health," *Journal of Trace Elements in Medicine and Biology* 28 (2014): 357–363, http://dx.doi.org/10.1016/j.jtemb.2014.09.002.

INDEX

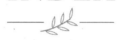

ABOUT THE AUTHOR

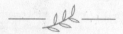

D r. Meredith Warner founded her Baton Rouge clinic, Warner Orthopedics and Wellness, in April 2013. Having served earlier in the US Air Force as a surgeon and in private practice since 2005, Dr. Warner understands how poor diet, stress, lack of restorative sleep, and lack of energy lower the body's ability to fight disease. The result of addressing these: prolonged recovery.

An expert in foot and ankle surgery and other orthopedic injuries, Dr. Warner wanted to open her own orthopedic clinic in Baton Rouge to better serve her patients and to expand the services she would be able to offer if she were hospital employed—services that treat the whole person and capitalize on the latest research about diet, natural treatments, and alternative methods to protect and heal the body with less-invasive procedures offered through traditional medical practices.

In addition to her orthopedic practice and wellness firms, she teaches physicians at Louisiana State University's Department of Orthopedic Surgery. Dr. Warner is also the inventor of The Healing Sole footwear and Well Theory, a breakthrough wellness protocol designed to empower people with the tools they need to treat their pain naturally, improve sleep, and extend their health span.